Praise for *True Wellness the Mind*

"*True Wellness the Mind* is a welcome ad   ...nce-supported integration of Eastern and Western medicine, presented in a well-documented yet very readable and motivational format. I have seen, experienced, and researched many of the benefits discussed by Drs. Kurosu and Kuhn. In a world becoming ever more stressful, *True Wellness the Mind* includes research that shows that mindful practice can actually change the structure of the brain, enhancing our ability to deal with stress and anxiety, and promote the healing ability of the body. Their work does an excellent job of incorporating Eastern modalities of healing with Western approaches to medicine, forwarding a new era of science-based holistic health. A must-read for anyone feeling frustrated with conventional approaches to health or who would like to explore broader avenues founded on several millennia of practice."

—Dr. Peter Anthony Gryffin, PhD, MS, author of *Mindful Exercise: Metarobics, Healing, and the Power of Tai Chi.*

"In the spirit of the biopsychosocial model in health psychology, *True Wellness the Mind* does a wonderful job of combining the very best of Western and Eastern practices to comprehensively address the biological, psychological, and social aspects of depression, anxiety, and sleep. The reader is presented with a thoughtful roadmap on how to address these life challenges. By showing the reader how to integrate Western and Eastern interventions, and highlighting the importance of self-healing, Drs. Kurosu and Kuhn provide us with valuable tools on our journey toward the overall goal of wellness."

—Claudette Ozoa, PhD, clinical psychologist, Honolulu, HI

"Depression, anxiety, and sleep challenges are the major issues that lead people to seek psychotherapy treatment. *True Wellness the Mind* offers readers not just a theoretical understanding of the combined power of Western and Eastern approaches to mental health issues, but also step-by-step instructions and tools to address mental health challenges. With accessible and practical suggestions, Drs. Kurosu and Kuhn support the reader in establishing small, meaningful behavioral changes, knowing that, ultimately, each of us can be an active participant in our own health."

—Warren R. Loos, clinical psychologist, PhD, Honolulu, HI

"Following up on their excellent book, *True Wellness*, which focused on ways to integrate Eastern and Western approaches to health care, Catherine Kurosu and Aihan Kuhn have put together a new volume focusing on the mind. *True Wellness the Mind* is, like its predecessor, a clear, balanced consideration of how we can benefit by choosing approaches from what the authors call the 'continuum of medicine.'

"The book is intended to assist readers in gaining a better understanding of the underlying causes of anxiety, depression, and sleep disorders, all of which can contribute to health issues. The authors hope to inspire readers to modify detrimental behaviors and learn to adopt beneficial practices, with the assistance of health-care providers. And, of course, they are advocating a complementary mix of Western and Eastern approaches.

"Kurosu and Kuhn are clearly proponents of the role that Eastern approaches can play in promoting well-being. What is refreshing, however, is the balance they bring to their discussion. They are not wide-eyed enthusiasts making overly broad promises for the benefits of arcane techniques from the Mystic East. On the contrary, the authors are well grounded in an understanding of and appreciation for the scientific method and Western medical practice. They are quite clear in stressing that they conceive of Eastern medical approaches as tools to be used only as complementary to, and to the extent they are compatible with, Western medical science. In this regard, they are careful to provide research citations that support their discussion—a welcome and rare practice in popular approaches to nontraditional medicine.

"In their exploration of a 'continuum of medicine,' the authors stress a need for cross-cultural understanding of medical approaches. They provide a cogent discussion of the history and philosophy of both Western and Eastern traditions. They note the tendency for Western medicine to fragment treatment into discrete areas of focus, contrasting this with more holistic Eastern approaches influenced by, for example, Daoism.

"Kurosu and Kuhn present a solid discussion of Western research that examines the effects of breath control and meditation on wellness and provide a fascinating (and honest) assessment of research completed to date on the efficacy (and mystery) of acupuncture.

"The writers are clearly proponents of the benefits of activities such as qigong and tai chi in health promotion. Their assertions on the benefits of such activities is less well grounded in research studies than other topics, but this is more a reflection on the state of scientific investigation than it is a failure on their part.

"To assist in activities that can help individuals with stress, anxiety, and insomnia, the work includes illustrated instructions on basic qigong exercises, helpful checklists for self-healing practice, self-assessment tools, and dietary guides. The authors have provided simple, clear tools for self-help that nicely supplement the more theoretical portions of the text.

"In short, *True Wellness the Mind* provides a well-thought-out, lucid, and concise resource on ways to integrate Eastern medicine with Western treatments. By providing a balanced presentation of research to date on aspects of Eastern medicine and a judicious emphasis on complementary integration of medical approaches, they have crafted a fine resource for those looking to expand their understanding of Eastern medicine, as well as a solid practical guide for individuals wishing to take the next step and explore the health benefits of this tradition."

—John Donohue, PhD, author, dan-ranked in Shotokan Karate-do, Kendo, Shinshin Ryu Iaijutsu

"*True Wellness the Mind* is a timely guide on how to use integrative therapies to treat the modern-day ailments of stress, depression, anxiety, and insomnia. Practitioners, healers, and wellness-seekers can all benefit from the wisdom of this book. Kurosu and Kuhn blend the best strategies of Eastern and Western medicine into clear and easy-to-follow steps that will allow readers to overcome emotional and physical barriers that may be standing in the way of optimal health."

—Valerie Cacho, MD, medical director of sleep medicine, Hawaiʻi Pacific Health: Straub Hospital, Honolulu, HI

"Catherine Kurosu and Aihan Kuhn's latest book, *True Wellness the Mind*, effortlessly blends Eastern and Western approaches to emotional wellness. It is intellectually rigorous in its explanations of the mind and how it works and yet readily accessible in its suggestions for daily cognitive and behavioral strategies to promote wellness. The authors draw from both traditions to provide a primer on how to get started on the path to emotional balance."

—Nancy Halevi, PsyD, licensed clinical psychologist, Kailua, HI

True Wellness the Mind: How to Combine the Best of Western and Eastern Medicine for Optimal Health by Drs. Kurosu and Kuhn is their second book on true wellness. This book focuses on healing anxiety, depression, and sleep disorders using a combination of Western and Eastern medicine. The authors do an excellent job of explaining the history, philosophy, and science of Western and Eastern medicine, as well as presenting the respective healing modalities for anxiety, depression, and sleep disorders. Then, the authors emphasize the benefit of qigong for anxiety, depression, and insomnia, with easy-to-follow, step-by-step practical instructions. At the end, the authors provide the True Wellness Checklist, with simple instructions to help readers get started.

"In *True Wellness the Mind*, Drs. Kurosu and Kuhn use evidence-informed, patient-centered care and therapeutic approaches for these complex health conditions. This book will benefit health-care providers by guiding them to help patients make better treatment choices, and benefit other readers by offering a better understanding of how integrative therapeutic approaches, combining Western and Eastern medicine, help in healing anxiety, depression, and sleep disorders. I will be implementing these approaches in my daily practice at work and home."

—Jo Ann Liu, DNP, AOCNP, University of Michigan Integrative Oncology Scholars 2018–2019, Duke Cancer Institute

"The doctors have published a very good body of work on an important yet challenging subject: integrative medical treatment for anxiety, depression, and insomnia. I have been practicing integrative medicine since 1997 and will be recommending *True Wellness the Mind* as necessary reading for patients who are dealing with these issues."

—Robert J. Schmidt, MD, LAc, Family Medicine BC, Clinical Lipidology, BC

"In this succinct yet thorough book, authors Catherine Kurosu and Aihan Kuhn present the history and philosophies of Eastern and Western medical modalities and provide practical applications for implementation of both in our hectic world today. When suffering from anxiety, depression, or insomnia, the brain's ability to conceive of solutions is diminished, and *True Wellness the Mind* offers feasible and immediately implementable methods for change. This integrative approach to wellness promotes an important paradigm shift for lasting recovery and healing."

—Gina Cargile, trauma model therapist, certified hypnotherapist, Reiki healer at Honolulu Acupuncture and Naturopathic Clinic, HI

CATHERINE KUROSU, MD, LAc
AIHAN KUHN, CMD, OBT

TRUE WELLNESS THE MIND

How to Combine the Best of
Western and Eastern Medicine for
Optimal Health; Sleep Disorders,
Anxiety, Depression

YMAA Publication Center
Wolfeboro, New Hampshire

YMAA Publication Center, Inc.
PO Box 480
Wolfeboro, New Hampshire 03894
1-800-669-8892 • info@ymaa.com • www.ymaa.com

ISBN: 9781594396649 (print) • ISBN: 9781594396656 (ebook)

Managing Editor: T. G. LaFredo
Cover design: Axie Breen
This book typeset in Minion Pro and Frutiger.

10 9 8 7 6 5 4 3 2 1

Publisher's Cataloging in Publication
Names: Kurosu, Catherine, author. | Kuhn, Aihan, author.
Title: True wellness, the mind : how to combine the best of Western and Eastern
    medicine for optimal health; sleep disorders, anxiety, depression / Catherine Kurosu,
    Aihan Kuhn.
Description: Wolfeboro, NH USA : YMAA Publication Center, [2019] | Series: True
    wellness. | Subtitle on cover: How to combine the best of Western and Eastern
    medicine for optimal health: sleep disorders, anxiety, depression. | Includes
    recommended reading and resources, and index.
Identifiers: ISBN: 9781594396649 (print) | 9781594396656 (ebook) | LCCN: 2019841777
Subjects: LCSH: Mental health. | Self-care, Health. | Alternative medicine. | Health
    behavior. | Sleep disorders—Alternative treatment. | Anxiety—Alternative
    treatment. | Depression, Mental—Alternative treatment. | Exercise—Psychological
    aspects. | Nutrition—Psychological aspects. | Stress management. | Acupuncture. |
    Qigong. | Mind and body. | Well-being. | Health—Alternative treatment. | Holistic
    medicine. | Medicine, Chinese. | BISAC: HEALTH & FITNESS / Sleep. | HEALTH
    & FITNESS / Healing. | HEALTH & FITNESS / Healthy Living. | SELF-HELP /
    Mood Disorders / Depression. | SELF-HELP / Self-Management / Stress
    Management. | MEDICAL / Alternative & Complementary Medicine.
Classification: LCC: RA790.5 .K87 2019 | DDC: 362.2—dc23

NOTE TO READERS
The practices, treatments, and methods described in this book should not be used as
an alternative to professional medical diagnosis or treatment. The authors and publisher of this book are NOT RESPONSIBLE in any manner whatsoever for any injury
or negative effects that may occur through following the instructions and advice con-
tained herein.

It is recommended that before beginning any treatment or exercise program, you consult your medical professional to determine whether you should undertake this course
of practice.

Printed in Canada.

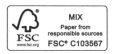

Table of Contents

Foreword by Jeanne Heroux, MSN   vii

Preface   xi

CHAPTER 1
Emotional Health, Sleep, and Disease   1

CHAPTER 2
The Continuum of Medicine   9

CHAPTER 3
The True Wellness Approach to Anxiety and
Depression   43

CHAPTER 4
The True Wellness Approach to Sleep Disorders   72

CHAPTER 5
Qigong for Anxiety, Depression, and Insomnia   99

CHAPTER 6
General Principles of Self-Healing   120

CONCLUSION   125

Acknowledgments   127
Recommended Reading and Resources   129
Glossary   131
Index   137
About the Authors   143

To our patients, past, present, and future

Foreword

EVERY SO OFTEN, SOMETHING MAGICAL HAPPENS. Think about the joyous ceremonial union of a seemingly unlikely couple. Here we are about to embark upon an extraordinary journey with the marriage of Western and Eastern medicine. Drs. Kurosu and Kuhn have artfully and scientifically blended these two traditions in *True Wellness the Mind*, the second book in their True Wellness series.

I have known Aihan Kuhn as a doctor, instructor, mentor, and, also, a friend for well over a decade. I've taught qigong since 2008, having learned from Dr. Kuhn the practical, mechanical science along with the positive, vital spirit of qigong and tai chi. I speak at her yearly Qigong / Tai Chi Healing Institute's annual conference in Sarasota. Dr. Kuhn trained in both Western medicine and traditional Chinese medicine. Early in her career, she trained in obstetrics and gynecology while in China. She uses various holistic methods such as traditional Chinese medicine, qigong, and tai chi for healing, Daoist healing, mindful eating, dieting, hands-on healing, and therapeutic exercises. Her mind/body medicine has helped many patients with amazing results.

I know Catherine Kurosu as an expert in her field as an OB-GYN and as an acupuncturist. She is an adventuresome spirit who brings a calming presence wherever she goes. Dr. Kurosu is trained as a medical doctor and practiced obstetrics and gynecology for almost twenty years, while also learning the benefits of acupuncture. She is now a diplomate of the American Board of Medical Acupuncture and the National Certification Commission for Acupuncture and Oriental Medicine. Both doctors have combined the expertise of their original training and broadened their scope of practice to include more holistic, preventative, and curative methodologies.

Recently, I had the profound honor and pleasure of spending four days with Dr. Kurosu, with Dr. Kuhn as our gracious hostess in her serene Sarasota home. We spoke together of the chasm between Eastern and Western approaches and how this gap has gradually been closing. I have found both psychiatry and obstetrics to be more open to alternative modalities than are more conventional medical fields such as, for example, cardiology and pulmonology. However, even these specialties have, over the past ten years, begun to value a more holistic approach to total wellness, as opposed to a single-minded focus on curing disease.

Some doctors recognize that drug treatments are not providing their patients with the long-term benefits they'd hoped to achieve. Patients continue to suffer with symptoms of their disease despite progressively stronger medications. Does medical intervention sometimes thwart the body's self-healing mechanisms, and even promote disease progression? Can nutrition and various natural, holistic therapies enhance the body's own response toward stress and dis-ease? Can a combination of Western and Eastern modalities achieve optimum wellness? If you have read this far, you may be thinking, "yes." And, you are right!

Do you ever wonder, if the natural approach is so effective, why aren't more doctors using it? While progress is being made, such as doctors increasingly recommending omega-3 fish oils or glucosamine sulfate for their patients, for example, the truth is, doctors are uncomfortable with recommending many of the myriad modalities available, primarily because they know only what they have been taught. The typical medical doctor who graduated nine or ten years ago had fewer than twenty hours of nutritional training during their four years of medical school and basically was given no mention, let alone a survey, of therapies such as herbal medicine or acupuncture. Fortunately, more recent graduates have been exposed to these healing modalities through courses in integrative medicine during their training.

I am a nurse practitioner, board certified in both medicine and psychiatry. Over the years, I have observed many disconnects in our allopathic medical and psychiatric fields: patients are looking for a "cure," but frequently can't tell me what medications they are on or what they take them for; the Western model strives to "fix" the patient by alleviating symptoms, but often ignores the underlying root cause of the disease; when providers *do* discuss the many stressors that contribute to a patient's illness, the patient may not be willing to make the recommended changes. Often, patients verbalize their preference for taking a pill to counteract the symptoms of stress, rather than reduce the stressor itself. I have found that lifestyle change can be a struggle for some, until it is too late. *True Wellness the Mind* emphasizes taking control of our own medical care, rather than outsourcing it to a medical provider. The authors suggest that we, ourselves, are responsible for our own mental and physical health, and provide easy-to-follow steps to true wellness.

I currently specialize in addiction medicine, but I have worked in hospitals for more than twenty years, including more than ten years in emergency departments. During this time, I have seen many examples of the ways stress manifests. My favorite example of people's anxiety-ridden response to stress occurred in the emergency room at least twice per month. A horrified patient is brought in by ambulance, believing they are "having a heart attack." They describe tremendous chest pain, sometimes radiating, shortness of breath, and nausea, all red flags for a potential cardiac emergency. Once all the test results are in, and it has been determined they are not going into cardiac arrest, they look at me with complete, utter perplexity and ask, "What happened?" And, "I still feel awful!"

At this point, I order a calming agent such as lorazepam for them, but long before that arrives, I take one of their hands in mine and say, "Just breathe with me." They dutifully comply, and together we breathe long, slow, deep, slender breaths. As we breathe together, their breaths become longer, until, after about three minutes, they became relaxed. Often they even refuse the lorazepam! I explain that they had worked themselves into a state of panic, a "fight-or-flight" response over some stressor, or an accumulation of them, and induced the symptoms of a heart attack. At this point, they often feel embarrassed. But, those are such great teaching moments! It is a chance to explain how the anxiety generated in our mind can completely derail our body, and, in turn, how our brain, with simple slow breathing, can invoke a parasympathetic response, gradually calming us down.

You will find the same types of "teaching moments" right here! Within the covers of this book are discussions of the connection between chronic stress and brain function/malfunction, the importance of sleep and how to optimize it, and a multitude of stress-reduction techniques, including qigong exercises, complete with explanatory illustrations and the wisdom of the Dao. A thorough, easy-to-understand explanation of acupuncture describes how utilizing the piezoelectricity of the entire body leads to a reduction of pain, stress, depression, anxiety, and more.

Drs. Kurosu and Kuhn also discuss behavior modification and lifestyle changes for managing factors that cause stress such as trauma, external and internal pressures, and emotional imbalances—conditions with which we all struggle if we live in modern society. There are a plethora of self-help and holistic therapy books out there, but I can guarantee you that none of them create the same effective fusion of East meets West as does *True Wellness the Mind*. So, read on and struggle no more!

Jeanne Heroux, MSN
Board Certified Psychiatric Nurse Practitioner
Board Certified Adult Medicine Nurse Practitioner
Owner of The Affinity House, A Sober Home for Women

Preface

WE LIVE IN AN EXTRAORDINARY WORLD. The technical advances of the past century are incredible, but they can also be overwhelming. In most parts of the world, life is fast paced, pressured, and nonstop. We are in constant communication with the society around us, including those on the other side of the globe. With cell phones, computers, and internet streaming, we are continually absorbing information regarding current events. These events can be inspiring, entertaining, or disturbing. They are always with us and available for viewing. Gone are the days when radio and television broadcasts stopped at midnight and resumed in the morning. Information overload is available every moment of the day or night.

And it is not just information that is accessible. Supermarkets, pharmacies, and restaurants provide twenty-four-hour service. No longer are emergency workers like police, firefighters, and medical personnel the only people who work nights. Checkout clerks, waitstaff, bus drivers, shelf stockers, and cleaners are among the many workers who are expected to pick up night shifts.

Between endless media interactions, longer working hours that disrupt the usual rhythm of the day, and the ever-present need to work faster and harder, we find our patients are increasingly stressed and sleep deprived. The demands that modern society places on us, and that we place on ourselves, are creating a situation in which we can never fully succeed. We worry that we have left work undone or that we have not attended to our families. We worry about our finances and our communities and the future. Indeed, many people have a lot to worry about— poverty, unemployment, illness, religious persecution, racism, violence, and war.

Such circumstances may naturally lead to emotional distress, but even for those who have a comfortable existence, constant worry can give way to anxiety, depression, and difficulty sleeping. We have seen among our own patients how chronic stress can wear away at their well-being, often by first stealing their sleep, then dampening their mood, and finally disrupting their health. Sometimes a sudden change can have such a negative effect on people's lives that startling, debilitating shifts occur in their emotional and physical health. Other patients seem to have a tendency toward psychological and sleep problems. Such patients may exhibit these features under "normal" conditions, and others may manifest these disorders only when exposed to external stressors.

Why are some people more resilient than others, even among those who have no genetic predisposition to such problems? How do some people keep themselves emotionally healthy even under extreme stress? How can people maintain restorative sleep under these circumstances? Modern researchers are attempting to answer these questions, but so many societal and environmental influences act on an individual that it is difficult to tease apart the answers. The circumstances are as different as each person's underlying constitution.

As physicians, when we encounter patients struggling with anxiety, depression, and sleep problems, we recognize that emotional health, physical health, and sleep are intertwined, each affecting the others. We work with our patients to help them identify adjustments they can make to optimize these three aspects of good health. Improvements in any area will act synergistically on the others and create a positive change.

Our purpose in writing this book is to help the reader understand the intricacies of anxiety, depression, and sleep disorders; modify behaviors that are detrimental; initiate practices that are healing; and seek assistance from a health-care provider to guide the reader's progress. It is our firm belief that readers who are troubled by these conditions should have a thorough evaluation by a Western medical professional. Eastern healing modalities may be used concurrently if they are compatible with Western care and administered by a qualified practitioner.

Modern science is unraveling the biological processes responsible for brain function. With that knowledge, we are learning how chronic stress not only affects our sleep and mood, but actually alters the structure and function of the brain. The brain can change, for better or worse. It is our hope that readers will use the Eastern and Western treatment approaches in this book to restore normal brain architecture and processing. With persistence, you can achieve emotional well-being and restful sleep.

Catherine Kurosu, MD, LAc
Aihan Kuhn, CMD, OBT

CHAPTER 1

Emotional Health, Sleep, and Disease

FOR MANY CENTURIES, humans have appreciated the connection between our emotional and physical health. Sleep lies at the interface between these realms, influencing and being influenced by our minds and bodies. When we find our mind troubled, our sleep disrupted, and our body out of balance, it is sometimes difficult to determine the initial cause.

This is like the classic question, "Which came first, the chicken or the egg?" When talking to patients about their medical history, a lot of information can be gained by trying to unravel the "chicken or egg" conundrum. When someone is asked, "When was the last time you felt well?" he will almost always know the month and year. The follow-up question, "What happened in your life during the previous few months?" can shed a lot of light on the problem. Some people have experienced an emotional trauma that has not resolved, leading to anxiety, depression, or difficulty sleeping. Subsequently, they develop physical ailments such as headaches, digestive issues, or chronic pain. Other people suffered a physical trauma that disrupted their sleep and led to anxiety and depression. The physical trauma could have been an accident or an illness, a surgery, or a lifelong disability.

Any initiating trauma, whether physical or emotional, can lead to disrupted sleep. This can be caused by the physiological changes brought about by a medical condition or by the worry and stress caused by a change that the initiating trauma has brought about in relationships or socioeconomic factors. For example, if someone is in a car accident and is injured, she may suffer both physical and emotional trauma. The physical injury may cause pain, disfigurement, or disability, which may result in an inability to work, either inside or outside the home. People injured in this way may be unable to care for their children, parents, or partner. Perhaps now they cannot financially support their family. This can lead to worry, anxiety, and depression. Individuals who are unable to fulfill their usual responsibilities commonly feel ill at ease in their relationships and society at large. These physical and emotional stressors can adversely affect a person's sleep. Not only can pain from a physical injury disrupt the normal sleep cycle, but the emotional strain of altered circumstances can also lead to insomnia. Head injuries, in particular, can disturb a person's normal brain function and sleeping pattern. The physical and emotional trauma caused by traumatic brain injury (TBI) can take years to resolve.

The example of a car accident is a common one, but any serious illness or life change can lead to emotional problems and sleep disorders. Some people are able to bounce back from these situations and get right back on course. Others, because of the severity of their injury or illness, never truly recover and may carry the secondary burden of poor sleep and emotional distress for the rest of their lives. Yet again, some people are genetically predisposed to suffer from emotional or sleep disturbances; such conditions are known to run in families. With increasingly sophisticated tests such as gene sequencing and functional magnetic resonance imaging of the brain (fMRI), and a greater understanding of how brain cells actually work, scientists are able to pinpoint the reason some people are affected with these disorders and others are not. For instance, generalized anxiety disorder carries a moderate genetic risk, with a 30 percent risk of inheritance.[1] A 2018 meta-analysis found

---

1. Michael G. Gottschalk and Katharina Domscke, "Genetics of Generalized Anxiety Disorder and Related Traits," *Dialogues in Clinical Neuroscience* 19 (2): 159–168.

44 genes that may predispose an individual toward major depression.[2] Continued research into sleep reveals that it is under genetic control. Sleep involves many layers of biochemical processes, and genetic abnormalities can account for various types of sleep disorders.[3] It is important to note, however, that the authors of these studies, and many more, point out that anxiety, depression, and sleep problems are significantly influenced by environmental, societal, and lifestyle factors. This means that even though a person's genetics might make them susceptible to these conditions, they may not actually experience any symptoms of these illnesses. In Western medicine we call this "gene expression." Whether certain genes are expressed depends on where, how, and with whom a person lives. If you live in a crowded, polluted area, if you suffer from loneliness and isolation, and if you eat poorly and rarely exercise, the genetic information stored in the cells of your body can be expressed in such a way as to allow some diseases to occur.

Even if you have been fortunate and have avoided a major crisis, like an accident or illness, the way you live your life day to day makes a significant difference to your health. One of the main contributors to good health is adequate restful sleep. Humans have always realized that sleep is important, but we are just starting to understand exactly why. We all know that when we sleep well, we wake up refreshed and energized. Our thinking is clear and our memory is sharp. We also know that the reverse is true. When we are sleep-deprived, we feel sluggish, our reaction times are slower, and we have difficulty with problem solving. In fact, one British study that compared sleep deprivation to alcohol consumption found that seventeen to nineteen hours without sleep resulted in the same level of performance on speed and accuracy testing as having a blood alcohol level of 0.05 percent. After twenty-three hours, the

---

2. Naomi R. Wray, Stephan Ripke, and the Major Depressive Disorder Working Group of the Psychiatric Genomics Consortium, "Genome-Wide Association Analyses Identify 44 Risk Variants and Refine the Genetic Architecture of Major Depression," *Nature Genetics* 50 (5): 668–681.

3. Amita Seghal and Emmanuel Mignot, "Genetics of Sleep and Sleep Disorders," *Cell* 146 (2): 194–207, https://doi.org/10.1016/j.cell.2011.07.004.

performance levels were the same as if a person had a blood alcohol level of 0.1 percent, which is well past being legally intoxicated.[4]

So why is sleep so important to the brain? What happens to our brain when we sleep? It gets cleaned. In the body, the system that removes the waste products of cellular metabolism is the lymphatic system. A fluid called lymph picks up these waste products and takes them through lymph vessels to the nodes and organs, such as the spleen, to be processed. But the brain does not have lymph vessels or nodes like the rest of the body. The equivalent of lymph in the brain is known as cerebrospinal fluid (CSF). The CSF carries the waste products of the brain cells; it was recently discovered that the way the CSF travels between cells deep in the brain is through spaces between the walls of the blood vessels and the projections of a type of brain glial cell called an astrocyte. Glial cells are not neurons. The various types of glial cells support the functioning of the neurons that make up your brain. So, instead of a totally separate system of vessels to transport waste products, as is found in the lymphatic system of the body, the brain uses the space between the outside of the blood vessel and the specialized glial cells to clear the brain of toxic by-products. Scientists have named these channels the glymphatic system, meshing the words "glial" and "lymphatic" to convey its function and form.[5]

This is all very interesting, but you may be thinking, "What does this have to do with sleep?" It turns out that the glymphatic system is incredibly active when we are asleep and is almost completely suppressed when we are awake. In order for harmful substances to be cleared from the brain, you must be asleep. If these toxic by-products accumulate in the brain, over time, diseases like Alzheimer's and other forms of demen-

4. A. Williamson and A. Feyer, "Moderate Sleep Deprivation Produces Impairments in Cognitive and Motor Performance Equivalent to Legally Prescribed Levels of Alcohol Intoxication," *Occupational and Environmental Medicine* 57 (10): 649–655, doi:10.1136/oem57.10.649.

5. N. A. Jessen, A. S. F. Munk, I. Lundgaard, and M. Nedergaard, "The Glymphatic System—A Beginner's Guide," *Neurochemical Research* 40 (12): 2583–2599, doi:10.1007/s11064-015-1581-6.

tia may occur. The glymphatic system may also distribute nutrients and neurotransmitters that keep the brain functioning normally. Since the activity of the glymphatic system is enhanced during sleep, it is no wonder that we need adequate amounts of sleep to feel alert and well rested on waking.

Even our mood improves after sleeping well. In fact, normal sleeping patterns are linked to normal mental health. Among people with illnesses such as depression, anxiety, bipolar disorder, or schizophrenia, sleep disturbances are common and may actually precede mental illness in susceptible individuals. Fortunately, because sleep and emotional well-being are so closely intertwined, improving sleep quality in such patients can decrease the symptoms of psychiatric illness by as much as 50 percent.[6]

Sleep is one of the principal resources you need to keep your body and mind functioning well. Along with nutritious food and a safe and supportive living environment, sleep is essential to maintain your equilibrium in life. Another word for this equilibrium is "homeostasis," your ability to sustain all the physiological processes your body needs to stay healthy and in balance.

Homeostasis or balance set points change over time and circumstances. Everyone has been through periods when life seems off-kilter. Maybe you had to sleep less or work harder to accomplish a goal. Perhaps you lost your job or got a promotion. You may have married, divorced, or lost a loved one. All these events may require you to use more of your resources—your time, your money, your strength. All these events and more are considered stressors. We have not even discussed environmental stressors such as pollution and overcrowding; societal stressors such as racism, gender bias, and poverty; and catastrophic stressors such as war, violence, and abuse. The word "stress" often has a negative connotation, but even normally joyful events, such as the birth of a baby, can be stressful.

---

6. Russell Foster, "Why Do We Sleep?" TED Talk, June 2013, http://www.ted.com/talks/russell_foster_why_do_we_sleep.html.

When you live through these stressful life events, changes occur in all aspects of your physiology. This "gearing up" to face the increased demands on your metabolism, intellect, or psyche has been referred to as "allostasis," meaning "achieving stability through change."[7] These stressors could be good, tolerable, or toxic. Whether "good" or "bad," the cumulative effects of such stressors are referred to as the "allostatic load."[8] Under usual circumstances, this state of heightened functioning resolves and your immune, endocrine, and nervous systems are taken off high alert. Ordinarily, we are able to cope with these periods of allostasis, especially if we have been attentive to the needs of our bodies and minds, staying healthy, active, and well rested. This is much like topping up your bank account, saving for the proverbial rainy day.

But not everyone has the same reserves. Your fiscal, physical, or emotional state can vary throughout your life. Sometimes uncontrollable events occur one on top of the other. Sometimes we simply do not take the time or make the effort to care for ourselves as we know we should. Whatever the reason, when stressors overwhelm your resources, the body and mind are unable to return to a state of homeostasis, or balance. In this condition, dysregulation of the immune, endocrine, and nervous systems occurs. Essentially, you get "stuck" in overdrive. This is called "allostatic overload," and it can create havoc.[9] Prolonged exposure to abnormal levels of immune modulators, hormones, and neurotransmitters results in physical changes throughout the body, leading to chronic inflammation and chronic diseases such as diabetes, heart disease, autoimmune conditions, pain syndromes, and psychological problems. In the brain, exposure to the biochemical profile produced by

---

7. P. Sterling and J. Ever, "Allostasis: A New Paradigm to Explain Arousal Pathology," in *Handbook of Life Stress, Cognition and Health*, edited by S. Fisher and J. Reason, 629–649 (New York: John Wiley and Sons, 1988).

8. B. S. McEwen, "Central Role of the Brain in Stress and Adaptation: Allostasis, Biological Embedding, and Cumulative Change," in *Stress: Concepts, Cognition, Emotion, and Behavior,* Handbook of Stress Series, volume 1, edited by G. Fink, 39–55 (New York: Elsevier, 2016).

9. Ibid.

allostatic overload can actually change its structure. Three brain regions affected by such toxic stress are the hippocampus, the amygdala, and the prefrontal cortex. These areas communicate with each other and modulate cognitive function, fear, aggression, and self-regulation. The interaction among these three regions also plays a part in turning on and turning off the neural and endocrine systems' response to stress.

The hippocampus is involved in memory of daily events, special memory, and mood regulation. The prefrontal cortex deals with decision making, working memory, and self-regulatory behaviors such as mood and impulse control. Both of these structures help shut off the stress response, but under prolonged allostatic overload, the brain cells in these regions shrink and some of the connections between other brain cells are lost, allowing the chemical mediators of toxic stress to continue.

In contrast, the amygdala is the portion of the brain responsible for the autonomic nervous system's response to memories and emotions, particularly involving fear, anxiety, and aggression. The amygdala turns on stress hormones and causes the heart to beat faster. Under chronic stress, the cells in the amygdala enlarge and create more connections among other brain cells, further driving the physical and emotional aspects of the fight-or-flight response.

By understanding how the architecture of the brain changes under chronic stress, you can see how difficult it can be to recover from a period of extreme stress. Sleep deprivation can make matters even worse. In people with depression or anxiety disorders, it is as though the nervous system is locked in this abnormal physiological state. Although it is tempting to rely solely on medications to correct this imbalance, numerous studies cite the effectiveness of the concurrent use of behavioral interventions to restore normal central nervous system activity and structure, as much as possible. Such interventions include physical activity, cognitive-behavioral therapy, meditation, and the cultivation of strong social support and integration.[10]

---

10. Ibid.

As we shall see in chapter 2, Eastern healing modalities such as meditation, tai chi, qigong, and yoga are able to transform the architecture of the brain and modulate the neuroendocrine-immune system to restore normal function, behavior, and sleep. By using effective treatments from both Eastern and Western traditions, you may see prompt and long-lasting improvements in your emotional and physical health. Although an understanding of the history and philosophy of Western and Eastern medical systems is not required to utilize their beneficial treatments, it will give you an appreciation of these approaches to patient care.

CHAPTER 2

The Continuum of Medicine

WHEN WE GET SICK, physically or emotionally, often the first questions we ask are how and why did this misfortune befall us? These questions have been asked for millennia. In ancient times, illness was attributed to the supernatural. Afflicted people thought they were being punished by a god, possessed by an evil spirit, or hexed by some malignant force. Various legends and myths were created in all societies in an effort to explain the how and why of disease. "Cures" were generally ritualistic and of a spiritual nature, administered by the "doctor" of the group. These healers went by different names in different cultures—shaman, curandero, kahuna—but they all blended their understanding of culture, community, and physical environment to create rituals and remedies to treat illness within their tribes.

Over time, as nature was better understood, the realization came that diseases were caused by real-world phenomena and not by supernatural forces. With this awareness came a shift in the role of the shaman. The shaman continued to be the spiritual leader of the group, but the physical health of the community was left to others—the herbalists, the bonesetters, and the surgeons who were the doctors of the tribe. Even though the shaman and the doctor now had different responsibilities, there remained a consistent understanding of health and healing. They knew that the health of an individual was more than the correct functioning of the body. True healing involved the patient's mental and emotional well-being. In many ancient traditions, doctors realized that to view their patient as a complete person, they had to consider all aspects of that patient's life; medical conditions, relationships within the family and community, and daily habits would all influence the quality and quantity of the patient's life-span. Those daily habits were, and still are, the cornerstone of health maintenance. These physicians encouraged adequate sleep, nutritious food, and exercise. Not only was physical exercise recommended, but mental discipline and quiet concentration of the mind were promoted for complete well-being of the body, mind, and spirit. Through these methods, the physician helped people maintain good health and recover from illness.

The following discussion of the history and philosophy of Western and Eastern medicines will shed some light on how and why doctors in each discipline approach patient care the way they do. We then discuss the science behind the Eastern healing arts and the current trend toward integrating these two medical systems.

The History and Philosophy of Western Medicine

The birthplace of Western medicine was ancient Greece, and its father was a physician named Hippocrates (460–360 BCE). Hippocrates felt that a clear understanding of the patient's way of life and constitution was essential in order to provide appropriate medical care. He particularly emphasized balance in daily living regarding food and exercise. In ancient Greece, the human body was thought to be composed of three material substances: blood, water, and bile. These substances were called "humors." Additionally, the humors were associated with certain qualities (hot, cold, moist, and dry) and elements (earth, air, fire, and water). Perfect health was considered to be the ideal equilibrium of the humors, qualities, and elements within each individual, and disease was the result of imbalance among these components.

Even prior to the birth of Hippocrates, Greek philosophers and physicians were fascinated with the natural world and, like the Chinese, used observations of their environment to explain human growth and development. It was thought that the universe consisted of pairs of opposite qualities, such as hot and cold, moist and dry. Harmony between these pairs was considered paramount, as an imbalance could result in disease. This principle of paired opposites is also seen in the Chinese theory of yin and yang, which we discuss below.

Another parallel between Eastern and Western medical thought was the concept of "vitalism." This is the notion that within the human body there is an active and intelligent force that instinctively maintains the health of the whole person. This "vital force" is similar to the Chinese concept of qi.

This idea of a dynamic energy within every individual was central to the art and science of medicine in Europe until after the Renaissance, during the Scientific Revolution (1450–1630 CE). During the Scientific Revolution, doctors were able to use advancing technology to examine the intricate workings of the human body and the environment. For example, in 1609, the light microscope was invented and, for the first time, doctors and scientists could see organisms that were invisible to the naked eye. They called such organisms microbes. Over the next two centuries, into the 1800s, an understanding of these organisms developed. It was proven that microbes, further classified as bacteria, viruses, or molds, could cause disease. Once it was known that specific organisms caused specific diseases, treatments were created that could cure many illnesses that previously resulted in severe disability or death. Over time, vaccines were invented that could prevent some diseases altogether. The study of microbiology and the development of antibiotics and vaccines are some of the most significant discoveries of Western medicine.

With this astounding success in the treatment of infectious disease, Western physicians realized that, if they could find the cause of an illness, they might be able to develop a cure. From this point onward, the study of medicine focused on the search for the simplest single explanation for the origin of a whole host of ailments. By the time the Industrial Revolution in Europe was in full swing, the study of medicine was influenced greatly by the societal changes of the era. Factories emerged, and every part of the production process was compartmentalized. No longer did an artisan see the creation of an item through from start to finish. Rather, a worker manufactured one portion of the item, then passed it on to the next worker and then the next, until completion. This preference for fragmentation became pervasive in Western medicine. Technology gave physicians and scientists the ability to break down biochemical and physiological processes into ever-smaller component parts. This has led to an unprecedented understanding of the complexity of the human body.

New discoveries are still being made: from the understanding that a person's constitution can be passed down to offspring to the complete mapping of the human genome, from realizing that living things are made up of cells to understanding how these cells function and how we can use modern medicine to change these processes. New drugs, new surgical techniques, and new therapies are continually being discovered, trialed, and then, if successful, offered to patients. One of the main difficulties of this explosion of knowledge is how to master it and implement it correctly. The production line increased efficiency during the Industrial Revolution, with each worker perfecting a certain aspect in the manufacturing process. Modern medicine has also undergone a similar division of labor.

With the increasing complexity of biomedicine, it has become impossible to know everything about the human body, how we get sick, how we heal, and all the possible therapeutic interventions that can be used for every possible illness. Medical students the world over gain basic knowledge in anatomy, physiology, and biochemistry, then branch out to learn about the many causes of disease and how to cure or improve a patient's condition. Upon graduating from medical school, young doctors in most countries are required to train further. They choose from many branches of medicine and become specialists in that field. Even doctors who want to become family physicians do a three-year residency in general medicine to hone their skills. Others choose from general surgery, internal medicine, obstetrics and gynecology, psychiatry, radiology, and pathology. After completing at least four years in their specialty, they can then subspecialize—they can focus on the medical or surgical aspects of every single body part or process. From the brain to the feet and everything in between, you can find a subspecialist to meet your needs.

But, even as a subspecialist, it is difficult to keep up with every new scientific discovery in the field. Subdividing and specializing medical research and care is a way of trying to achieve this impossible task. Similarly, the search for the single underlying cause of a particular disease is a way for modern medicine to develop treatments that hope to correct problems at the cellular, genetic, or molecular level of the body. In many instances, this approach has been spectacularly successful. For example, the discovery of the underlying cause of type 1 diabetes led to the discovery of insulin and methods to isolate it from animal sources and manufacture it synthetically, and now even to transplant the cells that create insulin and allow a diabetic to survive. Without the curiosity and ingenuity of physicians and scientists, this and other medical breakthroughs would not exist.

For many conditions, however, this reductionist approach has not been successful, or has even created more problems. The biomedical model of seeking out a solitary cause of an illness may overlook the possibility of interplay among many factors that can contribute to a disease. These factors can be specific to an individual, such as genetics, family environment, and personal life experience, or they can be factors that affect the community at large, such as environmental pollution, food additives, and poor access to markets with fresh produce or green spaces in which to exercise.

The dynamics of the origin of disease are highly complex, especially with respect to the chronic diseases of Western societies, such as heart disease, type 2 diabetes, autoimmune conditions, and some gastrointestinal disorders. For many of these conditions, the biomedical model may not be the best way to institute effective health care. A growing body of evidence suggests that optimizing the way we eat, move, think, and sleep can do more to reverse chronic illness than medications or surgery. Adopting such lifestyle changes may even prevent these conditions in the first place.

The importance of what we eat and our level of activity, sleep quality, and calmness of mind are not new concepts in medicine at all. In Western medicine, these concepts were vital millennia ago and are reemerging today. Increasingly, students of Western biomedicine are being trained to consider all aspects of an individual and their illness. This patient-centered model is called "biopsychosocial medicine." Practitioners who hold this viewpoint evaluate not just the biological cause of a disease but the psychological, emotional, spiritual, and socioeconomic factors involved. All these elements can both affect and be affected by the disease process. Through this understanding, more and more medical practitioners are able to help patients heal and maintain optimal health.

The History and Philosophy of Eastern Medicine

Before discussing the chronology of Eastern medicine, an appreciation of its philosophy is extremely important. The principles of Eastern medicine hinge on the concept that man is inseparable from the universe. This notion comes from the observations and practices of Daoism. Daoism is a philosophical system that was reportedly founded by Laozi (b. 604 BCE). Laozi formulated the tenets of Daoism, but it was his students and followers who wrote the majority of the formal texts that are the foundation of this philosophy. Prior to the advent of Daoism in China, as in every primitive civilization, the ancients observed the changes that took place over time in the world around them. They noted the cycles of the moon, planets, and stars. These celestial patterns were correlated to weather changes, growing seasons, and animal migrations. Daoism grew out of this naturalist school of thought as it attempted to understand man's place in the order of the universe. This law of nature is called "the Dao." In English, this translates as "the Way" or "the Path." The Dao represents the basic principles from which all phenomena follow, including all aspects of human behavior.

In addition to recording the ideas of the Dao and the phases in the physical world that change over time, Daoist thinkers helped formalize the concept of the unity of opposites within nature. This is the basis of yin-yang theory, for which Eastern medicine is known. By starting with the concept of opposition to describe the relationship between two entities, Daoists formulated a dynamic view of the world that could be used to explain universal processes. A classic example of this mode of thought is the observation that there is always a sunny side and a shady side to a hill, wherein one can say this side of the hill is sunny only by comparing it to the shady side. Labels are given to each item being described— as either yin or yang—depending on its degree of substantiality. If something is more passive and receptive in nature, it is yin; if it is more active and dynamic, it is yang. But these definitions have meaning only when compared one to the other. Any of the pairs that embody yin and yang cannot be separated and are not absolute.

The yin-yang experience is a fundamental factor in the development of the Daoist metaphysic. Far from designating yang as "something" and yin as "nothing," Daoism recognizes that both are active and that one creates the other.[1] For example, the ceramic of a teacup would be considered yang and the space within the teacup considered yin. It is the space that is filled and makes the ceramic useful as a teacup. The yin and the yang of the cup are inseparable.

From this thought arises the realization that the part and the whole must exist simultaneously. The infinite exists at every singular point in space, and eternity is found in every individual moment. The Daoist consideration of the infinite and the yin-yang experience infuses itself into the practice of Eastern medicine by virtue of the fact that dysfunction within the patient, known as the pattern of disharmony, cannot be viewed separately from the patient herself. The part and whole exist together and define each other.

In addition to the concepts of Dao and yin-yang, the recognition of the phases of the universe was developed into the theory known as Wu Xing, or Five Phases. Wu Xing has also been translated as Five Elements, however, many scholars state this is incorrect. The word "element" implies a component part or constituent ingredient. The word "phase" denotes a dynamic process. In his iconic book, *The Web That Has No*

---

1. Michael M. Zanoni, PhD, conversation with author (CK), April 10, 2011.

Weaver, Dr. Ted Katpchuk describes the Five Phases as patterns that occur in dynamic systems. Each phase has a designated name and displays a set of particular characteristics.[2] The phases are known as Wood, Fire, Earth, Metal, and Water. The names of the phases are not as important as each set of characteristic qualities and functions. Wood represents growth. Fire represents maximal growth that has reached its apex and will plateau or decline. Metal is emblematic of decline. Water denotes a profound state of rest that has reached its nadir and will shift toward growth or activity. Earth represents balance.[3] If you imagine a pendulum swinging to and fro, the Earth Phase would be the moment at which the pendulum is hanging straight down. The patterns of the Five Phases can be seen in the ebb and flow of all natural and even man-made phenomena: human growth, maturation, and decline; the changing of the seasons; economic expansion and recession; the rise and fall of political powers.

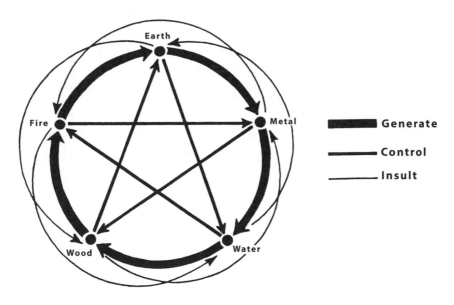

---

2. Ted J. Kaptchuk, OMD. *The Web That Has No Weaver: Understanding Chinese Medicine* (New York: McGraw Hill), 437.

3. Ibid., 438.

As long ago as the fourth century BCE, the Five Phases were used to understand and interrelate naturally occurring events. This understanding was applied to medicine as well as other disciplines, including astrology, social politics, and natural sciences.[4] Using this paradigm, Daoist physicians looked at the human body as a microcosm of the universe and sought to use the natural laws of the universe to maintain a harmonious balance. They acknowledged that this balance must occur internally and also with the patient's external environment. Following the principles of Daoism, which emphasize moderation and equilibrium, the patient would be cautioned to follow the middle path in all aspects of life: to rest but also exercise, to work but have time for leisure, to eat a variety of healthy foods but neither too much nor too little. By achieving this equilibrium, the movement of the intelligent vital force within the body (called qi) would be smooth. This free movement of qi would maintain optimal health.

In 1973, in the Chinese province of Hunan, a famous archeological dig discovered silk texts that discussed subjects as diverse as astrology, art, military strategy, philosophy, and medicine. There were even two copies of Laozi's *Dao De Ching*, found in the Mawangdui tombs (King Ma's Mound). Scientific methods were used to date the texts from approximately 200 BCE; the tomb itself had been sealed in 168 BCE. The medical texts cover physiology, illness, surgery, herbal treatments, and what has been translated as "macrobiotic hygiene." Macrobiotic hygiene involves not only the body but also the spirit; this section discusses longevity, sexuality, and diet. Breathing and physical exercises are recommended to treat illness and cultivate health, and there are also writings on magic and incantations.[5]

Illness is described in the Mawangdui medical manuscripts as the result of a disturbance in the movement of qi within the eleven vessels

---

4. Joseph Helms, MD, *Acupuncture Energetics: A Clinical Approach for Physicians* (Berkeley, CA: Medical Acupuncture Publishers, 1995), 17.

5. Donald J. Harper, *Early Chinese Medical Literature: The Mawangdui Medical Manuscripts* (London: Routledge, Taylor, and Francis, 1998), 6.

of the body. These vessels that contain qi are different than the arteries and veins that contain blood. The treatment that was advocated at the time involved cauterization of the qi vessels. There is no mention of using acupuncture needles to correct the flow of qi. Instead, the medical practitioners who wrote these manuscripts advocated the use of food, herbs, breath control, and exercise to improve the flow of qi and achieve a long and vibrant life.

This approach to good health was formalized in the classic medical text of the Han dynasty (206 BCE–220 CE), the *Huang Di Nei Jing* (*The Yellow Emperor's Classic of Internal Medicine*). It is thought that this text is a compilation of medical writings from practitioners of earlier centuries, which takes the form of a discussion between the Yellow Emperor (Huang Di) and his minister; it is significant in that it was the first known text to move away from shamanism and supernatural causes of disease. Like the Mawangdui medical manuscripts, the *Huang Di Nei Jing* discusses the prevention and treatment of illness through diet, exercise, and herbs. Acupuncture theory is well described in the second volume of this text. The principles of energy flow within the body (qi), yin-yang theory, and diagnostic techniques are also discussed.

Around the first century BCE, the art of acupuncture using metal needles was formalized. Some researchers of Chinese medical history state that acupuncture arose from the practice of using sharpened stones and bones to lance infected skin, allowing the body to heal. However, scholars such as Donald Harper and Paul Unschuld state that the vessel theory and treatment paradigm delineated in the Mawangdui medical manuscripts was the necessary precursor to acupuncture theory as described in the *Huang Di Nei Jing*.[6]

Through trial and error, the Chinese determined that placing acupuncture needles at specific sites would give consistent and reproducible results. By the time the *Huang Di Nei Jing* was written, the intricate system of acupuncture points and qi flow within acupuncture channels

---

6. Ibid., 5; Paul U. Unschuld, *Medicine in China: A History of Ideas* (Berkeley, CA: University of California Press, 1985), 95.

The Body Channels

Two Centerline Channels
Conception Vessel (Con)
Governing Vessel (Gov)

Twelve Principal Channels
Stomach Channel (Sto)
Spleen Channel (Spl)
Small Intestine Channel (SmI)
Heart Channel (Hea)
Bladder Channel (Bla)
Kidney Channel (Kid)
Pericardium Channel (Per)
Triple Warmer Channel (TrW)
Gall Bladder Channel (GaB)
Liver Channel (Liv)
Lung Channel (Lun)
Large Intestine Channel (LaI)

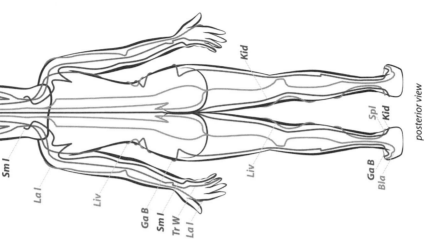

posterior view

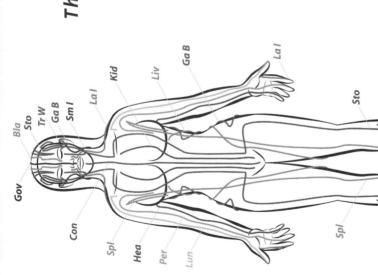

anterior view

Illustration courtesy of Shutterstock

was well established. Twelve paired principal channels, or vessels, were described, meaning that the channels were duplicated on each side of the body in a mirror image. These paired channels are named for organs of the body. The channels are kidney, heart, small intestine, urinary bladder, spleen, lung, large intestine, stomach, liver, *san jiao*,[7] pericardium,[8] and gallbladder.

The channels can directly influence the named organ, but they also affect other areas and physiological processes. Additionally, eight "extraordinary" channels are noted. These special channels run in various directions, over and through the body, connecting the principal channels and acting as reservoirs of qi. Acupuncture theory is discussed in more detail later in this chapter.

As in all ancient civilizations, the Chinese used indigenous plants, minerals, and animals as medicine. Chinese herbology predates acupuncture, probably by thousands of years, but until the development of written language the use of these medicinals was not documented. Several very famous texts categorize Chinese herbs and explain their function. *Shen Nong Ben Cao Jing* (*The Divine Farmer's Materia Medica*) was written in the early Tang dynasty (452–536 CE), but it is actually a compilation of much earlier writings. The book discusses the attributes of 365 herbs, the majority of which are still used today.

Dr. Zhang Zhong Jin (150–219 CE) was renowned for his text, the *Shang Han Lun* (*Treatise on Cold Damage*). This is the oldest formulary to group patient symptoms into clinically useful categories. Zhang Zhong Jin was also the first to link diagnoses derived through the principles of yin-yang theory and the Wu Xing (Five Phases) with standardized herbal treatments.

One of the most celebrated physicians in the history of Chinese medicine was Dr. Li Shi Zhen. He lived during the Ming dynasty and in 1578 wrote his masterpiece, the *Ben Cao Gang Mu* (*Compendium of Materia Medica*). Li Shi Zhen traveled across China in search of

---

7. Also known as Triple Heater or Triple Burner.
8. Also known as Master of the Heart.

medicinal herbs. After twenty-seven years of diligent work, the *Ben Cao Gang Mu* was completed. It documents 1,892 distinct herbs and more than eleven thousand formulas. This comprehensive text remained the official materia medica for China for the next four hundred years.

Two other noteworthy Chinese doctors are Hua Tuo (145–203 CE) and Sun Si-Miao (581–683 CE). Hua Tuo was well known, especially for his surgical skills and the development of a particular type of exercises that he called Five Animal Play (Wu Qin Xi). Sun Si-Miao stood out not only for his talent as a healer, but also for his humanity. Although the emperors of the Tang dynasty wanted Sun Si-Miao as the palace physician, he declined and worked for all people. In his writings, he instructed doctors to be of good moral character and to treat all patients equally, regardless of their class or wealth.

Around the time of Sun Si-Miao, during the fifth and sixth centuries, Eastern medicine spread from China to Japan, Korea, and Vietnam. Through trade via the Silk Road, knowledge of this system of medicine eventually arrived in the Middle East and Europe, with little more than passing interest outside Asia until much later. As European colonization of East Asia increased, more Western physicians became curious about these techniques. France had colonized Vietnam, and so French physicians who traveled there were exposed to the successes of acupuncture and herbal formulas. From the eighteenth century onward, the French were at the forefront of Western investigations of Eastern medicine. Later in this chapter, we discuss the science of acupuncture and other Eastern healing modalities in greater detail.

An increasing percentage of the general population has benefited from Eastern medicine over the past century, but in the United States very few were able to take advantage of this powerful medical system prior to the 1970s. Until then, acupuncture was illegal in America. Even though it was practiced and well respected throughout Europe, Britain, Canada, Japan, and other Asian countries, both practitioners and patients who sought to use this medicine risked arrest in the United States. For this reason, very little documentation remains of the early history of Eastern medicine in America; there are, however, some accounts dating as far back as the nineteenth century. In 1974, California became the first state to legalize the practice of acupuncture, after which most other states began to follow suit. Acupuncture training and credentialing became more formalized, but a few states still remain in which there is no acupuncture practice act to regulate the profession. In all states except Hawai'i, a medical doctor or osteopath may practice acupuncture, for which most states require approximately three hundred hours of acupuncture training; such a practitioner is called a medical acupuncturist. A licensed acupuncturist who is not a physician will have completed approximately three thousand hours of training in acupuncture and herbology. This also would include hundreds of hours of Western biomedicine such as anatomy, biology, chemistry, physiology, and pharmacology.

Whether a medical or licensed acupuncturist, the mark of an excellent practitioner is the willingness to refine the art and science of Eastern medicine. Collaboration between acupuncturists and other healthcare practitioners is happening more frequently in clinics, hospitals, and academic institutions. The drive to comprehend the mechanism of action of acupuncture, qigong, tai chi, yoga, and meditation has fueled thousands of basic research studies and clinical trials. In the discussion that follows, we provide a brief summary of the current understanding of how these therapies can heal the human body.

The Science behind Eastern Healing Modalities

From Asia to Europe to the rest of the world, interest in and use of Eastern medicine has grown during the past century, surging over the last fifty years. Several components of Eastern medicine have been subject to scientific scrutiny in the West, but also in their countries of origin. The elements of Eastern medicine (including Indian, Tibetan, and Chinese practices) that have been most researched are meditation and breath control, yoga, qigong, tai chi, herbal remedies, and acupuncture.

Regulation of the breath has been used for millennia to calm the mind and heal the body. Even without a modern understanding of how the brain and body communicate, the ancients formulated breathing techniques that balanced the autonomic nervous system. This is the part of your brain, nerves, immune, and endocrine systems that determines your state of relaxation. The autonomic nervous system is composed of the sympathetic nervous system and the parasympathetic nervous system. The sympathetic nervous system initiates the release of stress hormones when your brain perceives that you are in danger. These hormones cause your heart rate to elevate, your blood pressure to rise, and make glucose available to fuel your muscles in preparation for combat or evasive maneuvers. This reaction is known as the fight-or-flight response. In contrast, the parasympathetic nervous system calms all these processes and returns the body to a normal state of activity. Slow, deep breathing stimulates the main nerve of the parasympathetic nervous system called the vagus nerve, which in turn releases hormones and neurotransmitters that slow your heart rate, lower your blood pressure, and generally bring your body into balance.[9] The benefits of calming the nervous system include decreasing chronic inflammation, thereby decreasing your risk of chronic illness.

Controlling the breath is often one of the first steps employed in meditation. There are many different types of meditation—Buddhist, Hindu, Zen, Tibetan, Daoist, mindfulness, and many more. Depending on the ideology associated with the practice, the goals of meditation can range from relaxation and stress relief to compassion and spiritual enlightenment. Meditation usually results in a sense of calmness and clarity that can be difficult to describe. Numerous medical benefits have

---

9. T. M. Srinivasan, "Pranayama and Brain Correlates," *Ancient Science of Life* 11 (1/2): 1–6; D. Krshnakumar, M. R. Hamblin, and S. Lakshmanan, "Meditation and Yoga Can Modulate Brain Mechanisms that Affect Behaviour and Anxiety," *Ancient Science of Life* 2 (1): 13–19, doi:10.14259/as/v2i2il1.171; Michael M. Zanoni, "Healing Resonance Qi Gong and Hamanaleo Meditation," https://www.mikezanoni.com /meditation-qi-gong (accessed February 4, 2018).

been attributed to meditation, and scientists are investigating how meditation affects the brain and overall health.

When a person meditates, the electrical activity in the brain changes. This is true of any change of state such as intense concentration or emotion, drowsiness, sleep, and dreaming. These patterns of electrical activity are called brain waves and are measured by electroencephalography (EEG). Brain waves, also known as neural oscillations, have different frequencies. In addition, a wide range of patterns, combinations of frequency and amplitude are associated with different stages of sleep and wakefulness. For instance, you can be awake and in a state of deep concentration as you are trying to solve a problem or you can be awake but daydreaming and inattentive. Each of these states of wakefulness has different patterns involving each of the frequencies, but in different proportions, and can involve different areas of the brain. Simply stated, the higher frequency brain waves are associated with cognitive processing and alertness (beta waves). Lower frequencies are associated with sleep (delta waves). In between are frequencies associated with wakefulness (alpha waves) and deep relaxation, daydreaming, and meditation (theta waves). Combinations of delta and theta waves are important in memory processing. The state of mind between alpha and theta waves is said to be one of increased creativity.

Through the use of functional magnetic resonance imaging (fMRI), researchers have discovered that meditation increases the amount of gray matter in the brain, which is made up predominantly of the cell bodies of neurons,[10] and also seems to slow the natural loss of gray matter that occurs as we age.[11] Depending on its location within the brain, gray matter is involved with a variety of functions such as learning, mem-

10. Britta K. Holzel et al., "Mindfulness Practice Leads to Increases in Regional Brain Gray Matter Density," *Psychiatry Research* 191 (1): 36–43, doi:10:1016/j.pscychresns.2010.08.006.

11. N. Last, E. Tufts, and L. E. Auger, "The Effects of Meditation on Grey Matter Atrophy and Neurodegeneration: A Systematic Review," *Journal of Alzheimer's Disease* 56 (1): 275–286, doi:10.3233/JAD-160899.

ory, emotional regulation, and perspective. It seems that meditation can actually keep your brain younger and calmer.

A meditative state can be achieved during qigong, tai chi, and yoga. All these practices incorporate slow deep-breathing patterns, which confer all the benefits of seated meditation. These forms of moving meditation have additional advantages. During these practices, we move in well-defined patterns, stretching all the muscles in the neck, torso, arms, and legs. Stretching has many benefits, such as decreasing pain, improving blood circulation, increasing range of motion, and improving balance. For some time now, the cellular changes that occur with stretching have been studied. Dr. Helene Langevin and her team at Harvard demonstrated that by gently stretching the connective tissue of mice, inflammation at a site of injury was reduced. There was also an increase in the concentration of resolvins, which are cellular mediators that help coordinate the resolution of the acute inflammatory episode.[12] Later, using a similar rodent model and injecting breast cancer cells into the mice, Dr. Langevin found that gentle connective tissue stretching enhanced the response of the immune system and slowed the tumor growth by half.[13] This finding may offer an explanation for why many researchers have noted a lower risk of death from all causes, including recurrence, in cancer patients who exercise.[14]

An additional benefit of slow-moving, breath-focused exercise relates to the way the body utilizes oxygen. Dr. Peter Anthony Gryffin has compared the amount of oxygen in the blood during and after aerobic exercises like running and slow, mindful exercises like tai chi and qigong. It was previously known that the amount of oxygen in the blood, a measurement called blood oxygen saturation, either stays the same or

---

12. L. Berrueta et al., "Stretching Impacts Inflammation Resolution in Connective Tissue," *Journal of Cellular Physiology* 231 (7): 1621–1627, doi:10.1002/jcp.25623.

13. L. Berrueta et al., "Stretching Reduces Tumor Growth in a Mouse Breast Cancer Model," *Scientific Reports* 8 (2018): 7864, doi:10.1038/s41598-018-26198-7.

14. David O. Garcia, PhD, and Cynthia A. Thomson, PhD, RD, "Physical Activity and Cancer Survivorship," *Nutrition in Clinical Practice* 29 (6): 768–779, doi:10.1177/0884533614551969.

goes down during aerobic exercise as oxygen is being utilized by the large muscle groups, heart, and lungs. During slow-moving, breath-focused exercises, blood oxygen saturation initially goes up, then drops significantly for a short period of time before it returns to baseline. Dr. Gryffin's research suggests that this drop in blood oxygen saturation represents increased oxygen metabolism and diffusion throughout the whole body, since no excessive strain is placed upon the muscles and cardiovascular system as it is during aerobic exercise. Because of this unique difference in oxygen metabolism, Dr. Gryffin coined the term Metarobics to describe exercises that are neither aerobic, like running or swimming, nor anaerobic, like weight lifting. Metarobic exercises include tai chi, qigong, yoga, and other forms of moving meditation. This improved oxygen metabolism may account for many of the health benefits realized by practitioners of tai chi and qigong, such as decreased levels of chronic inflammation, improved immunity, and enhanced healing.[15]

Along with meditation, breath regulation, and movement, herbs are a mainstay in Eastern medicine, as well as in every medical tradition around the world. The healing properties of plants have been known for thousands of years, but not until the last two hundred years have specific biologically active compounds been extracted and used as drugs. As technology advanced, the medicinal properties of herbs were documented, particularly in China, where sophisticated combinations of herbs are used alongside modern pharmaceuticals in clinics and hospitals that integrate Western and Eastern care. The constituent components of these herbs, the ways they are metabolized, and how they affect the body continues to be documented. These plants have naturally occurring compounds that, depending on the herb, can act as antibacterials, antivirals, antifungals, hormone modulators, neurotransmitters, anti-inflammatories, antidepressants, or sleep aids. It is not within the scope of this book to discuss the biochemistry of all the herbs available to a qualified practitioner, but it should be noted that many of the formulas

---

15. Peter Anthony Gryffin, PhD, *Mindful Exercise: Metarobics, Healing, and the Power of Tai Chi* (Wolfeboro, NH: YMAA Publication Center, 2018), 15.

around today have been prescribed effectively in Asia for more than a thousand years.

The concept of using plants as medicines was well established throughout the world, but it was the mystery of acupuncture that fascinated the French. This led to various scientific experiments that laid the foundation for modern acupuncture research.

During the mid-twentieth century, the French and the Chinese performed a number of experiments that began to explain how acupuncture works. There is no single, simple explanation for acupuncture's mechanism of action. Each scientist added new information, helping to fill in the pieces of the puzzle.

In the 1940s and 1950s, Niboyet designed a series of experiments that showed electrical resistance is lower at acupuncture points than elsewhere on the body. This means electricity will pass into the body more easily across the skin at an acupuncture point than across the skin at a non-acupuncture point. Niboyet also demonstrated that electricity flowed more easily along the same acupuncture channel than between channels that were not as strongly related to each other. These results were confirmed by other scientists in the 1960s and 1970s.[16]

The acupuncture channel itself has remained an elusive entity. Our understanding of acupuncture channels and how acupuncture works has changed over time. Acupuncture channels are intimately associated with the neural, immune, and endocrine systems of the body. For example, modern acupuncture researchers note the channels that run on the inner arms almost exactly follow the paths of the nerves. Though the ancient Chinese were aware of the existence of the structures we call nerves, they did not know their function. They could not have known that electrical signals travel along nerves, having no knowledge of electricity.

Understanding that the effect of acupuncture is mediated via electricity was the first step in uncovering its mechanism of action. Over the past half century, the unfolding of this knowledge began by seeking

---

16. Joseph Helms, MD, *Acupuncture Energetics: A Clinical Approach for Physicians* (Berkeley, CA: Medical Acupuncture Publishers, 1995), 21.

evidence that these channels do exist. They were thought to be different than the known vascular or neurological systems that have been defined by modern medicine. The first piece of indirect evidence of the existence of acupuncture channels is that many patients experience a feeling of heaviness, achiness, or warmth around the acupuncture needles during treatments. These sensations can radiate from the needles, either circumferentially or linearly. When moving linearly, this feeling of warmth or achiness travels up or down the area of the body being needled. Modern Chinese researchers call this phenomenon "propagated sensation along channels."[17] They suggest that this sensation represents the movement of a corrective signal to an area determined by the acupuncture point that has been used. The target zone for the propagated sensation need not be a local area. Needling particular points on an arm or leg can reproducibly create a response in another part of the body. For example, certain points on the hand can alleviate back pain, a point on the lower leg can decrease discomfort of the opposite shoulder, and a well-known combination of points can initiate labor. We do know that the sensations elicited by acupuncture are an essential part of the signaling process and are caused by the activation of different types of nerve fibers.[18]

The speed of the propagated sensation has been noted to travel at one to ten centimeters per second. This velocity varies among subjects and with the intensity of the needling. This rate is much, much slower than the speed of nerve impulses, so it cannot be attributed simply to nerve conduction. The brain itself may also be involved in the perception of this sensation. Some studies have reported that amputees who are aware of phantom limbs are able to feel the propagated sensation within the absent limb when needled along a channel associated with the limb in question. This indicates that there must be some central nervous system involvement in the appreciation of this sensation.

---

17. Ibid., 22.

18. Michael Corradino, *Neuropuncture: A Clinical Handbook of Neuroscience Acupuncture*, 2nd ed. (London: Singing Dragon, 2013), 24.

When an acupuncture point is needled, a lot happens on the cellular level. There seems to be another mechanism at play, aside from direct activation of the nervous system. When the needle is inserted, it is manipulated to create sensation. This manipulation causes a mechanical change in the tissue. Researchers have demonstrated, using magnetic resonance imaging and ultrasound elastography, that a slow-moving wave is generated through the tissue that has been needled. There is also a shift in calcium ions that creates a biochemical signal that appears to be separate from the electrical signal of the nerve fibers.[19]

Western science has added a great deal of supporting evidence for the existence of a communication network from acupuncture points to the rest of the body by documenting the effects of acupuncture on blood chemistry, body temperature, and hormone levels. With respect to blood chemistry, acupuncture has been shown to modify levels of glucose, cortisol, triglycerides, and cholesterol. Although the mechanism of action is not well understood, acupuncture seems to assist the body in achieving balance. In medicine, this equilibrium is called homeostasis.

Acupuncture has also been shown to cause an increase in the body's surface temperature. This is caused by the dilation of vessels, resulting in increased blood flow. The increase has been documented at a rate three times higher than that of pretreatment flow. Not only does the surface temperature of the needled skin increase locally, but it also increases at the same area on the other side of the body.[20] Increased blood flow improves oxygenation within the tissue and may speed healing.

A great deal of research has been performed regarding acupuncture's effect on hormone and neurotransmitter levels, particularly with respect to pain relief. Some of these neurotransmitters include serotonin, norepinephrine, substance P, GABA (gamma-aminobutyric acid), and

---

19. Edward S. Yang et al., "Ancient Chinese Medicine and Mechanistic Evidence of Acupuncture Physiology," *European Journal of Physiology* 462 (2011): 645–653, doi:10.1007/s00424-011-1017-3.

20. Joseph Helms, MD, *Acupuncture Energetics: A Clinical Approach for Physicians* (Berkeley, CA: Medical Acupuncture Publishers, 1995), 40.

dopamine. All these compounds work together to diminish the brain's perception of pain.

Another way pain is decreased is through the release of cortisol, which has an anti-inflammatory action. The release of cortisol is controlled by levels of adrenocorticotrophic hormone (ACTH), and acupuncture has been shown to increase the discharge of this substance.

Finally, acupuncture modulates the body's internal production of opioids, leading to pain relief through a different pathway. Opioids are narcotic-like compounds; those produced in the body are called endorphins, which attach to receptors located on cell membranes, resulting in decreased pain. There are several different types of endorphins, and each acts at a different site within the brain and spinal cord to relieve pain. Interestingly, it appears that certain endorphins (beta-endorphin and met-enkephalin) also interact with the immune system. A surge in the levels of these endorphins can lead to increased activity of natural killer cells, a type of white blood cell that defends the body from foreign microbes and cancerous mutations.[21]

For all the various effects that acupuncture produces, the specific mechanism of action has not yet been completely discovered. As we have seen, electricity is a principal mediator of information that is passed along through the body, creating numerous physiologic changes.

Several theories exist regarding the ways in which these processes are regulated. Most concentrate on the effects produced by the passage of electrical current through the body. There is no doubt that the human body utilizes electricity in its everyday functioning. Western medicine has used this information to create many diagnostic tests and therapies.

In the heart, the interpretation of the electrical signals seen on an electrocardiogram (EKG) allows a physician to diagnose a heart attack or cardiac rhythm disturbance. If a patient's heart suddenly stops beating, electricity is applied to the person's chest via a device called a defibrillator in an effort to "kick-start" cardiac activity. Smaller amounts of electricity are also used to change irregular rhythms to regular ones.

---

21. Ibid., 41.

The electrical signals from the brain can be studied to help diagnose epilepsy or sleep disturbances. We can assess the health of these systems by recording the speed of electrical impulses through the nerves and muscles.

Even skin healing, which we tend to take for granted, requires electricity to activate the restorative process. Electrically, the skin can be described as a battery, with the negative charge inside each cell and the positive charge on the exterior surface. When the skin is breached, either by trauma or by inserting an acupuncture needle, the "battery" is short-circuited, and now the charge on the skin surface is negative. This negative charge seems to be an initiating factor in healing and activates the body's system of repair. It has been shown that this negative charge, described by Dr. Robert Becker as a "current of injury," can last several days following an acupuncture treatment.[22]

Dr. Becker, an American orthopedic surgeon, performed a fascinating series of experiments involving electrical current and limb regeneration in salamanders and frogs. Even though salamanders and frogs are closely related, salamanders can spontaneously regrow lost limbs, but frogs cannot. Through his research, Dr. Becker discovered that the tissue over the salamanders' limb stumps displays a relatively negative charge compared with other points on the animal. The frogs did not exhibit this negative charge. When he applied the appropriate electrical current and created a negative charge over the area of the frogs' missing limbs, the frogs' limbs regenerated just like the salamanders' did.[23] Dr. Becker's work has led to the creation of electrical devices that accelerate bone healing. These devices are used in cases in which broken bones are not healing well. In the past, it was sometimes necessary to amputate limbs that would not heal. By using electricity to enhance bone healing, Dr. Becker's discovery has decreased the need for amputation in such circumstances.

---

22. Ibid., 67.

23. Richard Gerber, *Vibrational Medicine: The #1 Handbook of Subtle-Energy Therapies*, 3rd ed. (Rochester, VT: Bear and Company, 2001), 91.

As well as the electrical component of the energy within the human body, there is also a magnetic constituent. Without this, magnetic resonance imaging (MRI) would not be possible. Studies called functional MRIs are used to observe the electromagnetic changes within different areas of the brain in response to acupuncture needling.

Other devices have been developed that can measure electromagnetic fields that come from diverse parts of the body. Such devices have demonstrated that electromagnetic fields exist around acupuncture points and that the intensity of these fields changes following acupuncture treatment.[24] Some researchers suggest that acupuncture points act as amplifiers by increasing the signal that moves along the channel.

Identifying the exact tissues through which these electromagnetic signals pass is a subject of ongoing study. Evidence suggests a variety of mechanisms through which bioelectrical information is transmitted. These mechanisms include the following:

- Electron-rich fluid that naturally bathes the tissues of the body, organized into tiny pockets now recognized as the interstitium, a newly defined organ[25]
- Perineural cells (cells that are adjacent to nerves)
- Proteins such as hormones and neurotransmitters that regulate communication between cells
- The fascia, a fibrous tissue that surrounds and connects every component of the body, from nerves, arteries, and veins to each muscle and organ

In his superb book *The Spark in the Machine,* Dr. Daniel Keown explains the role that fascia plays in the body, including its electrical properties. Fascia is composed of collagen. Collagen is a protein that accounts for

---

24. Joseph Helms, MD, *Acupuncture Energetics: A Clinical Approach for Physicians,* 1st ed. (Berkeley, CA: Medical Acupuncture Publishers, 1995), 62.

25. Petros C. Benias et al., "Structure and Distribution of an Unrecognized Interstitium in Human Tissues," *Scientific Reports* 8 (2018): Art. no. 4947, doi:10.1038/s41598-018-23062-6.

30 percent of the proteins in our body. Proteins are made of amino acids. In collagen fibers, these amino acids are arranged into three threads that twist around each other like three-stranded rope, lending incredible tensile strength to the tissues in which it is found. These include bones, ligaments, tendons, cartilage, arteries, and connective tissue. Just as it sounds, connective tissue connects and surrounds all our organs and muscles. Collagen even creates the lattice of the interstitium and interacts directly with the fluid inside these bundles, potentially allowing communication between body systems.[26]

Dr. Keown explains that, because of its molecular structure, collagen can act like a crystal and generate small currents of piezoelectricity when it undergoes mechanical stress. If a substance is piezoelectric, it will generate a change in electrical charge when it is compressed then returns to its original shape. We take advantage of piezoelectricity when we use pilot lights on a gas grill to create a spark, igniting the flame. Collagen is also a semiconductor, meaning that collagen can conduct electricity, but not as well as a metal such as copper. It can also act as an insulator, but not as well as glass. So, with every movement you make, your tendons, muscles, and bones undergo mechanical strain, and the collagen generates an electrical current. Collagen is an integral part of the fascia that connects the top of your head to the tip of your toes. Dr. Keown describes this as "an interconnected, living electrical web."[27]

When an acupuncture needle is inserted into the body, it makes contact with this "living electrical web." The acupuncturist will usually manipulate the needle until both the patient and the practitioner are aware of a certain sensation. The patient may feel an ache or a slight electrical zing at the insertion site, and this feeling may propagate along the body part that is needled. The acupuncturist can feel this through the needle. This sensation is called "de qi," or "the arrival of the qi." Even if the needle is inserted into an area that is not classified as an acupuncture

---

26. Ibid.

27. Daniel Keown, *The Spark in the Machine: How the Science of Acupuncture Explains the Mysteries of Western Medicine* (London: Singing Dragon, 2014), 21.

point or is not along the channel, this sensation may be felt. This is because the fascia wraps the whole body, not only along acupuncture channels. Just as the blood flows through large vessels and tiny capillaries, so too does piezoelectricity traverse the whole body.

Knowing about the "body electric," researchers have tried to explain the location of acupuncture channels and points, forming hypotheses regarding the way in which bioelectromagnetic information travels through the body. Zhang and Popp theorize that electromagnetic energy travels in waves. These waves bounce off the physical structures in the body such as bones, nerves, and skin, creating interference patterns, similar to the way waves of water reflect off the sides of a pool. As they change direction, the waves combine with others, creating higher waves, or canceling each other out. Zhang and Popp suggest that acupuncture points and channels occur at areas where bioelectromagnetic waves have combined to form new waves of higher amplitudes, and that acupuncture needles can be used to change the body's electromagnetic field.

Acupuncture needles may influence the state of the body through more than one single path. The human body is a complex system, and it seems likely that the ways in which acupuncture affects it are manifold. In an effort to tease apart the specific mechanism of action, researchers over the years have designed studies comparing true acupuncture with different sorts of pretend acupuncture, called sham acupuncture.

Sham acupuncture has been variously described as needling prescribed points superficially, needling non-acupuncture points, needling points that have not traditionally been used for the condition being treated, or using retractable needles to simulate the experience of true acupuncture without the actual needle insertion.

In numerous studies, sham acupuncture has been shown to be almost as effective as true acupuncture. Those that doubt the usefulness of acupuncture interpret this as placebo effect; however, whether using shallow needling, alternate points, or retractable needles, the collagen in the connective tissue of the body is still compressed. The piezoelectric property of collagen is activated whenever these tissues are compressed and microcurrents of electricity are generated. The body's response to the energetic input of sham acupuncture may not be as pronounced as when the points are actually needled, but the body responds nonetheless. This explains why, in some studies, sham acupuncture can be more effective than no treatment and almost as effective as "real" acupuncture, particularly if the sham acupuncture involves skin penetration. One interesting finding in a recent systematic review of acupuncture trials in the treatment of several types of chronic pain is that penetrating sham acupuncture more closely approximates the pain-relieving effect of true acupuncture than does the non-penetrating sham.[28]

Prior to today's clearer understanding of the physiological effects of acupuncture, many considered the improvements patients experienced to be the result of the placebo effect, which has been seen in medical practice for centuries. The word "placebo" comes for the Latin meaning "to please." The idea was that a doctor would give a patient a pill or treatment that was inert. If a pill, there was no active substance in it; if a treatment or surgery, there was no actual intentional repair of any structure. In spite of this inertness, a large number of patients actually improved or were cured. Historically, placebos have been used to encourage the patient's expectation that they would recover. From a research standpoint, placebos are used in an effort to ensure that the experience that both the study group and control group undergo is as close to the same as possible. This is done in an effort to isolate the one active substance or intervention that is creating a change in the patient's condition. Introducing a placebo group into a randomized controlled trial is a common occurrence, but as we have seen, sometimes placebos confuse rather than clarify the results.

Even when a study involves a simple cause-and-effect response, such as testing a new drug, it is impossible to separate the human reactions of the participants, both patients and researchers. Medical anthropologists, such as Claridge and Helman, have pointed out for some time that

---

28. A. J. Vickers et al., "Acupuncture for Chronic Pain: Update of an Individual Patient Data Meta-Analysis," *Journal of Pain* 2018 May;19(5): 455–474. doi: 10.1016/j.jpain.2017.11.005. Epub 2017 Dec 2.

there is a "total effect" of a drug or intervention that goes beyond the actual biochemical or physiologic nature of the treatment. The components that make up the total effect include the characteristics of the drug or treatment itself (even down to the color of the pill), the characteristics of the patient (age, gender, genetics, education, experience, personality, expectations), the characteristics of the researcher (personality, age, gender, attitude, professional status), and the setting in which the study is taking place.[29]

None of the above attributes can be removed from the clinical trial, and all of these characteristics are present within the study and placebo groups. This may, in part, explain why some patients who receive the active substance experience a negative clinical response and some within the placebo group improve.

So, does this mean that the positive clinical results experienced by placebo group patients are a figment of their imagination? No. In many studies, the improvements seen in the placebo group can be objectively identified. These changes are not just qualitative, meaning the patient describes a state of improved health. The differences can also be measured quantitatively, such as findings of lower blood pressure and lower cholesterol levels, and the decreased use of painkillers.

How can these changes be occurring? There is a great deal of interest in the physiologic effects of the placebo. Around the world, researchers are documenting changes that occur in the immune system, the brain, the spinal cord, and the biochemical balance of the body in response to a placebo.

In many of these studies, patients are not told they are receiving a placebo. For many health professionals, this presents an ethical dilemma in the use of placebos in general practice. Interestingly, at Harvard's Pro-

---

29. Elisabeth Hsu, "Treatment Evaluation: An Anthropologist's Approach," in *Integrating East Asian Medicine into Contemporary Health Care*, edited by Volker Scheid and Hugh MacPherson, 234 (Edinburgh: Churchill Livingstone/Elsevier, 2012).

gram for Placebo Studies, Dr. Ted Kaptchuk and others created a randomized controlled trial to look at the feasibility of using placebos without deceiving the patient.[30] All the patients had irritable bowel syndrome (IBS). The patients were randomized either to the open-label placebo group or the nontreatment control. Both groups received the same amount of time, counseling, and attention. Both groups were asked not to change any aspect of their usual routines for the duration of the study, such as starting a new diet or exercise program. Both groups had stable disease. The difference came at the end of the first interview, when the patients found out to which group they were assigned. The open-label group was told the pills they would take were "placebos, made of an inert substance, like sugar pills, that have been shown in clinical studies to produce significant improvement in IBS symptoms through mind-body self-healing processes."

The truly fascinating outcome of Kaptchuk's study was that even though patients knew they were taking placebos, their IBS symptoms improved more than those of the control group, which did not receive any pills. The statistically significant changes in the control group were decreased symptom severity and increased symptom relief. There was also a trend toward improved quality-of-life scores at the end of the study period for those taking placebos. Remember that these patients knew there was no medication of any sort in their pills, and yet they felt better. This demonstrates that the power of the mind to heal the body is astonishing. Eastern medicine has always recognized that fact and uses it to full advantage by incorporating meditation, qigong, and tai chi into patient care. Further research will shed light on this intriguing phenomenon. Even though the mechanism of action is not fully understood, we can still benefit from the positive physiologic changes that acupuncture and mind-body interventions produce.

---

30. T. J. Kaptchuk et al., "Placebos without Deception: A Randomized Controlled Trial in Irritable Bowel Syndrome," *PLoS One* 5 (12): e15591, doi: 10.1371/journal.pone.0015591.

Western Health-Care Providers and Eastern Medicine

Conventionally trained physicians all over the world are seeking ways to help their patients move toward optimal health. There is a strong sense among Western health-care providers that pharmaceutical and surgical interventions may not be enough to correct the course of modern diseases, the majority of which are caused by poor lifestyle choices. There is no doubt that under certain circumstances, medications and surgery can be lifesaving; however, medicine often does not get to the root of the problem and acts only as a temporary fix. Increasingly, doctors, physician assistants, and nurse practitioners recommend integrating complementary therapies into regular medical care.

Even without the input of a health-care provider, people are choosing to use supplements, herbs, and treatments that are not considered standard in Western medicine. The National Institutes of Health (NIH) regularly conduct surveys of tens of thousands of adults regarding their use of complementary or alternative medicine; approximately one-third of those surveyed use these therapies. Western practitioners now commonly ask their patients if they are using any other supplements, herbs, or alternative healing modalities. In fact, medical students are now taught to ask these questions as a matter of course, and academic health centers for integrative medicine can be found in such prestigious schools as Harvard, Tufts, Stanford, the University of Toronto, and the Mayo Clinic, to name but a few. Medical students are now learning about other traditional health systems so they can understand how these treatments can be safely integrated into conventional care. Hospitals are also offering non-allopathic healing services. The American Hospital Association released a survey in 2011 demonstrating that 42 percent of their member hospitals provided these modalities, representing an increase from 37 percent in 2007.[31]

---

31. American Hospital Association, "More Hospitals Offering Complementary and Alternative Medicine Services," September 7, 2011, https://www.aha.org/press

These complementary therapies cover a wide range of options and healing systems. Depending on practitioners' interests and experience, they may suggest adjunctive Western therapies such as biofeedback, relaxation techniques, massage therapy, health coaching, and lifestyle medicine programs. Or they might consider Ayurvedic medicine that incorporates yoga, meditation, herbs, and dietary therapies based on the patient's underlying constitution. Yet again, they may refer their patients to a practitioner of Eastern medicine. Like other healing systems, Eastern medicine is composed of various strands: dietary therapy, exercise, qigong, tai chi, meditation, bodywork, herbal formulas, and acupuncture. All these complementary therapies are aimed at improving the physical, mental, and emotional health of the patient and modifying underlying behaviors that contribute to chronic disease.

Many medical practitioners and patients will have preferences regarding which therapeutic intervention to use. After discussing the options, they may decide to stick with one traditional system entirely or mix and match depending on circumstances. For example, someone may respond well to Ayurvedic dietary therapy but have mobility problems and find it too difficult to get down on the floor to practice yoga. That person might do better with tai chi or qigong. Both of these Eastern practices will improve strength and balance as well as provide the preparation for meditation that yoga confers.

We too have our preferences. Our training in both Western and Eastern medicine has shown us that these two systems work extremely well together, and we are not alone. Over the span of two decades, the percentage of Western physicians who have a favorable opinion of Eastern medicine has increased fourfold. In 1998, only 20 percent of respondents held a positive view of Eastern medicine; when the survey was repeated in 2009, that number had exploded to 80 percent![32]

-releases/2011-09-07-more-hospitals-offering-complementary-and-alternative -medicine- services.

32. From the keynote address of the 2011 American Academy of Medical Acupuncture Symposium, given by Emmeline Edwards, MD, director of the Division of

Even the US military has embraced a component of Eastern medicine. In 2007, the US Air Force asked Dr. Joseph Helms, the founding president of the American Academy of Medical Acupuncture, to develop acupuncture protocols to treat conditions commonly found in combat veterans: post-traumatic stress disorder (PTSD) and pain, both acute and chronic. From 2008 to 2013, the US Department of Defense funded medical acupuncture training for hundreds of military doctors under the guidance of Dr. Helms. When this funding was no longer available, Dr. Helms created the Acus Foundation, a not-for-profit charitable organization, to continue training military health-care providers in medical acupuncture. Acus partnered with Nellis Air Force Base, training all the primary care physicians so that any patient could receive an acupuncture treatment at any visit upon request or recommendation. In the first year of this pilot program, opioid prescriptions dropped by 45 percent, muscle relaxant prescriptions decreased by 34 percent, and $250,000 was saved because of fewer referrals to civilian pain-management specialists.[33]

Although you may not have access to a primary care provider who is also a skilled acupuncturist, you can rest assured that a great many Western physicians are genuinely interested in incorporating Eastern therapies into conventional medical care. Your doctor may already know a number of reputable practitioners of Eastern medicine and would be happy to refer you. Some patients are reluctant to bring up the topic of incorporating Eastern medicine into their usual treatment plan. They are worried that they will offend their doctors. In this day and age, with all the emerging evidence demonstrating the effectiveness of acupuncture, meditative practices, and lifestyle changes, most physicians are open to adding these strategies to regular care. If your doctor *is* offended, we respectfully suggest you find a new primary care provider.

Extramural Research at the National Center for Complementary and Integrative Health, a component of the NIH, March 2011.

33. Acus Foundation, https://acusfoundation.org/our-programs/teaching/ (accessed June 13, 2018).

You will not know how your doctor feels about integrating Eastern and Western medicine until you have the conversation. As we discussed in our first book, *True Wellness*, there may be several reasons that your primary care provider has not spoken to you about these modalities. It may be that your doctor doesn't know whether Eastern medicine would be useful for your particular condition. Or she may not have access to reliable practitioners of Eastern medicine to whom she can send you. Or she may not want to suggest a therapy that might incur additional costs to you if your health insurance doesn't cover these services. These reasons should not prevent you from discussing treatment options with your doctor.

To have a meaningful discussion, you should come to the appointment prepared. You need to do a little homework. Since the inception of the internet, most physicians are very comfortable with patients who have done some online research about their illness and are happy to go through the downloaded information with you. If you are going to present your doctor with such information, it is important that it has come from reputable sources. The World Health Organization report on acupuncture is a good place to start. You could also search the websites of several prominent medical centers that offer Eastern medical services and see what conditions they commonly treat.

You should call your health insurance company to see whether Eastern medical services are a covered benefit and, if so, which providers are in the network. If this option is unavailable to you, you can cover the expense yourself, understanding that within three to five treatments you will know whether they are beneficial. If you live near a school of Eastern medicine, there will be a community clinic where you can receive care for a reduced cost.

Now that you have determined for yourself whether Eastern medicine is a suitable modality for your condition and how you can access that care, you will feel more comfortable broaching the subject with your doctor. Generally, the situations in which patients explore options outside of biomedicine are those in which the patient is not improving. In cases where the problem is acute, Western treatment options usually solve things quickly. For patients with chronic conditions, healing may be slower and require greater effort on the part of the patient and the physician. This is particularly true for patients who suffer from anxiety, depression, or sleep difficulties. Often both parties become frustrated with what appears to be a lack of progress. Eastern medicine is well suited to treating people in such circumstances. As we have mentioned previously, some patients do worry that their doctor would be offended at the suggestion of a complementary therapy but, in truth, that rarely happens. In our experience, most Western practitioners are interested only in their patients' well-being and are delighted at the prospect of successful treatment through Eastern medicine.

Occasionally, in difficult cases where a patient has not improved with conventional treatments, a physician may feel a sense of failure or embarrassment that she has not been able to help that person sufficiently. Following an honest and respectful discussion of Western and Eastern treatment options, often doctors and patients alike are relieved that a new plan has been formulated. Although the Western physician may not be administering the Eastern treatment herself, she would still be a part of your health-care team and would certainly do her best to facilitate this new aspect of your care where possible.

Finally, it is very important that you keep your doctor aware of any non-allopathic treatments that you are undergoing. Even if you have decided on your own to seek the help of an Eastern medical practitioner, your Western doctor needs to know this, particularly if you are taking any herbs or supplements. Many medications can interact with herbs, supplements, and foods, leading to dangerous situations in which the actions of drugs are either accentuated or diminished, resulting in medical complications.

Keep in mind that acupuncture and herbs, while extraordinarily effective, are not the only components of Eastern medicine. Acupuncture and herbs are treatments given to you by a skilled professional. But healthy food, moderate exercise, and a quiet mind are the foundation of Eastern medicine as well as many other healing traditions. Although both your Western and Eastern health-care providers can offer you encouragement and effective strategies for improving your physical and emotional well-being and sleep, only you can enact these changes to achieve optimal health.

CHAPTER 3

The True Wellness Approach to Anxiety and Depression

AN INCREASING NUMBER OF AMERICANS suffer from anxiety disorders and depression, either separately or in combination. Many other conditions, such as obsessive-compulsive disorder or posttraumatic stress disorder, can encompass some of the symptoms of anxiety and depression, but it is beyond the scope of this book to discuss them all.

It is estimated that more than 18 percent of the population suffers from some form of anxiety disorder,[1] and 10 percent of Americans report varying degrees of depression to their doctors.[2] The overlap is considerable, as almost half of individuals suffering from depression are diagnosed with a coexisting anxiety disorder.[3] Symptoms of generalized anxiety include worry, tension, agitation, sleep disturbances, fatigue, poor concentration, restlessness, and irritability. Those with depression can also suffer from all these symptoms, as well as depressed mood, decreased interest in life, diminished appetite, low self-esteem, and suicidal thoughts.

---

1. http://www.adaa.org/about-adaa/press-room/facts-statistics (accessed April 29, 2014).

2. http://www.cdc.gov/features/dsdepression/index.html (accessed April 29, 2014).

3. http://www.adaa.org/about-adaa/press-room/facts-statistics (accessed July 20, 2016).

Why some people become depressed or anxious and others do not is poorly understood. When subjected to similar life circumstances, one person may become severely affected, another may experience mild symptoms, and yet another may navigate the situation easily. Every individual has unique genetic and environmental predispositions toward depression or anxiety. With the inevitable stressors and losses we all encounter, some vulnerable individuals will develop alterations in the way their central nervous system functions. This, in turn, will change the body's biochemistry, resulting in symptoms of anxiety or depression.

Historically, the symptoms of both anxiety and depression were thought to be caused by abnormal neurotransmitter levels, so medications were developed to restore brain biochemistry to a more normal profile. For those who suffer from debilitating anxiety or are severely depressed, pharmacologic therapy can be very beneficial and even life-saving; however, drugs may not be as useful for other types of depressive disorders. If you suffer from milder forms of depression, you may receive greater benefit with fewer side effects from other modalities such as exercise, dietary changes, supplements, and mind-body techniques. These modalities can be used in conjunction with psychotherapy and pharmacotherapy, or both, after discussion with your health-care provider. Special attention must be paid to the use of supplements, herbs, or dietary changes if you are already taking any sort of antidepressant. These complementary therapies may affect the absorption, metabolism, or excretion of your current medication, resulting in unwanted side effects or serious complications.

It is worth noting that prescription medications may cause depression. A 2018 study published in the *Journal of the American Medical Association* (*JAMA*) highlights the link between depression and prescription medications. More than 26,000 people were surveyed, with 37 percent found to be using medications with depression as a known potential side effect. The authors found that the greater the number of medications used that listed depression as a possible side effect, the greater the likelihood the person would suffer from depression. Compared with people who used a similar number of medications that did *not* carry the risk of depression, and excluding people who took antidepressants, those who used at least three prescription medications with depression listed as a potential adverse effect were *three times* more likely to report symptoms of depression.[4] When designing the study, the authors did control for risk factors that might predispose patients to depression or suicidal thoughts, such as unemployment, poverty, and particular medical conditions. The authors found equivalent percentages of patients in each group were of the same socioeconomic class, were unemployed, and had similar medical conditions.

The authors of this study found more than two hundred medications that list depression or suicidal thoughts as potential adverse effects of the drug. Here are the categories of medications cited in the study, with a partial list of specified drugs within each category:

- Analgesics (painkillers like ibuprofen, hydromorphone, tramadol, oxycodone)
- Anticonvulsants (such as carbamazepine, clonazepam, diazepam, gabapentin)
- Antidepressants (including fluoxetine, paroxetine, selegiline, sertraline, bupropion, citalopram, trazodone, imipramine)
- Antihypertensives (blood pressure medication such as atenolol, enalapril)
- Anxiolytics, hypnotics, and sedatives (alprazolam, doxepin, zolpidem)
- Corticosteroids (cortisone, methylprednisolone, prednisone)
- Gastrointestinal agents (cimetidine, esomeprazole, metoclopramide, omeprazole)
- Hormones/hormone modifiers (finasteride, estrogens, progesterones, testosterone, anastrozole, tamoxifen)

---

4. Dima Mazen Qato, PharmD, PhD, Katharine Ozenberger, MD, and Mark Olfson, MD, MPH, "Prevalence of Prescription Medications with Depression as a Potential Adverse Effect among Adults in the United States," *JAMA* 319 (22): 2289–2298, doi:10.1001/jama.2018.6741.

- Respiratory agents (montelukast, ribavirin, cetirizine)
- Other therapeutic classes (interferon, cyclosporine, isotretinoin, baclofen)

It is startling to note that antidepressants can cause suicidal thoughts or depression, in fact worsening the very condition they are supposed to treat. Also, many other drugs listed are now easily available over the counter.

These findings demonstrate the importance of determining the underlying cause of a person's depression, whether polypharmacy is a main contributor, and whether management of concurrent medical conditions could be treated with other medications or lifestyle changes that would decrease the risk of depression as a side effect.

If you are concerned that your medications are adversely affecting your emotional health, speak to your health-care provider. If you have symptoms of depression, particularly if you have ever considered harming yourself or others, you should seek medical attention as soon as possible and before implementing any complementary therapies.

Regarding anxiety, the ADAA (Anxiety and Depression Association of America) commissioned a study in 1999 to look at how much of the US budget for mental health was consumed by anxiety disorders.[5] It turned out that $42 billion was spent on anxiety disorders. This represented about one-third of all expenditures on mental health. More than half of that $42 billion was used investigating the physical symptoms of anxiety that can be confused with other conditions. For example, palpitations can occur with anxiety but also can be a symptom of a heart condition. Patients with anxiety disorders are more likely to seek medical attention or be hospitalized than those without such conditions. Anxiety can mimic the symptoms of many diseases, but the reverse is also true: comorbid physical or mental illness can also exist at the same time within the same patient with an anxiety disorder. These illnesses can trigger each other, and it is often

---

5. P.E. Greenberg et al., "The Economic Burden of Anxiety Disorders in the 1990s," *Journal of Clinical Psychiatry* 60 (7): 427–435.

difficult to determine which came first. The following is a partial list of medical conditions in which anxiety can be a component:

- Headaches
- Irritable bowel syndrome (IBS)
- Sleep disorders
- Substance abuse
- Chronic pain
- Stress
- Eating disorders
- Heart disease
- Endocrine disorders
- Respiratory problems
- Neurologic conditions
- Menopause

Clearly, it can be difficult to tease out the predominant problem. Is the patient suffering from a medical condition of which anxiety is a symptom? Or is the patient suffering primarily from anxiety, the physical symptoms of which can copy those of other diseases?

There are many different types of anxiety disorders. The most common is called generalized anxiety disorder (GAD). Other sorts of anxiety stem from such conditions as obsessive-compulsive disorder (OCD), post-traumatic stress disorder (PTSD), social anxiety disorders, panic disorder, and phobias. The common thread among them all is that the patient cannot stop feeling anxious, worried, or panicked over certain thoughts that are, at times, illogical. Often these involuntary thoughts will completely disrupt the patient's life to the extent that he is unable to carry out daily activities. Anxiety disorders can interfere with all aspects of life, both at home and at work. In fact, many people turn to alcohol or drugs to relieve their feelings of anxiety. Some statistics quote alcohol abuse as high as 30 percent in those who suffer from panic disorders.[6]

6. Roberta A. Lee, MD, "Anxiety," in *Integrative Medicine*, 3rd ed., edited by David Rakel, MD, 122 (Philadelphia: Saunders/Elsevier, 2012).

Generalized anxiety disorder is defined as intense worrying that occurs on most days for more than six months, continually. Additionally, the patient must also have a minimum of three other symptoms or signs from the following list: trouble concentrating, trouble sleeping, tires easily, often irritable, restless, or has complaints of muscle tension.

The biomedical cause of generalized anxiety disorder is not yet clearly understood, but it appears that one of the areas of the brain is intricately involved: the amygdala. The amygdala is quite a primitive part of the brain of both humans and animals. One of its responsibilities is to relay information about dangerous situations to the autonomic nervous system. The nervous system then prepares the body to either fight or flee. Either response involves elevated levels of stress hormones that increase blood pressure and heart rate and create a heightened awareness of one's surroundings. This mechanism is perfectly normal and appropriate when a real danger is present. Anxiety disorders arise when a person repeatedly experiences these physiologic changes in situations that are not truly perilous. The memory of real danger cannot be erased from the amygdala, so the fight-or-flight response can easily be triggered in those who have suffered through traumatic situations such as war or physical abuse. Such patients are said to have post-traumatic stress disorder (PTSD). Still others have symptoms of anxiety without any inciting cause. In such people a genetic component may be involved that leads to an abnormal balance of neurotransmitters. This imbalance would cause a feeling of being in danger, disproportionate to the real situation at hand.

Regardless of the actual cause of anxiety, an integrative approach to treatment can be very effective. After seeking medical attention to rule out any underlying disease, you can use a combination of Eastern and Western treatment options to alleviate your symptoms. The "correct" approach will vary with each individual, as everyone has unique circumstances. It may be a matter of trial and error before you realize which combination of modalities serves you best. Discuss your situation, thoughts, and expectations with your health-care provider regarding these different approaches. As with any condition, consult your doctor before adjusting any medications you may be taking.

We now examine the Western and Eastern approaches to generalized anxiety disorder and depression. These interventions may also be appropriate for other anxiety disorder subtypes such as PTSD or OCD, but each should be vetted by your physician. If you are also suffering from depression or suicidal ideation, an immediate psychiatric evaluation is imperative.

Western Treatment Approach to Generalized Anxiety Disorder and Depression

Exercise

Many studies have documented the beneficial effects of exercise on generalized anxiety disorder and depression.[7] As we have discussed, exercise and diet can positively influence your brain chemistry, altering levels of dopamine, norepinephrine, serotonin, and endorphins, which can result in improved mood.

In fact, many studies have demonstrated that regular exercise is as effective as medication or psychotherapy in treating mild to moderate depression. If you are already in psychotherapy, taking antidepressants, or both, regular exercise should be incorporated into your treatment regimen. Exercising most days of the week will result in a higher level of well-being than drugs or psychotherapy alone.

With respect to exercise and anxiety, it seems aerobic activities such as running or swimming confer greater relief of anxiety than do weight training or stretching routines.[8] Therefore, it is important to perform

---

7. Brendon Stubbs et al., "An Examination of the Anxiolytic Effects of Exercise for People with Anxiety and Stress-Related Disorders: A Meta-Analysis," *Psychiatry Research* 249:102–108; T. Christian North, PhD, Penny McCullagh, PhD, and Zung Vu Tran, PhD, "Effect of Exercise on Depression," *Exercise and Sport Sciences Reviews* 18 (1): 379–416; Craig Schneider, MD, and Erica A. Lovett, MD, "Depression," in *Integrative Medicine*, 3rd ed., edited by David Rakel, MD, 92 (Philadelphia: Saunders/Elsevier, 2012).

8. Roberta A. Lee, MD, "Anxiety" in *Integrative Medicine*, 3rd ed., edited by David Rakel, MD, 123 (Philadelphia: Saunders/Elsevier, 2012).

some exercise that will elevate your heart rate. It appears that how long you engage in cardiovascular exercise is crucial to decreasing anxiety. This benefit was observed when the aerobic exercise session exceeded twelve minutes and peaked at forty minutes.[9] You don't necessarily need to start off at forty minutes of aerobic exercise daily. You can start slowly and work your way up to that level. Even if you exercise most days of the week and are able to include at least twelve minutes of aerobic activity, you should experience a decrease in anxiety-related symptoms.

No matter the form of aerobic exercise that you choose, regular exercise is definitely a mood enhancer!

Nutrition

Regarding nutrition, various modifications can improve anxiety[10] and depression.[11] Increased consumption of omega-3 fatty acids will improve serotonin metabolism. Serotonin is the main neurotransmitter thought to influence mood. Low levels of serotonin have been associated with both anxiety and depression. The omega-3 fatty acids play a crucial role in brain cell membrane and receptor function, allowing efficient processing of many neurotransmitters, including serotonin.

You can boost your omega-3 fatty acid intake by eating cold-water fish three times a week. If you don't like to eat fish, you can use fish-oil supplements. Also, flaxseed oil or ground flaxseed can confer a similar result. A Mediterranean-type diet will be rich in omega-3 fatty acids as well as encourage an increased intake in wholesome, unprocessed foods. If you prefer to use a supplement to ensure you get enough omega-3 fatty acids, start with one gram daily. The dose can be increased up to five grams per day.

Some foods should actually be decreased rather than increased. This applies to caffeine and alcohol. Caffeine is found in coffee, tea, energy drinks, and some soft drinks. It can increase your blood pressure and

---

9. Ibid., 123.
10. Ibid., 125.
11. Wendy Kohatsu, MD, "Nutrition and Depression," *Explore* 1 (6): 474–476.

heart rate and lead to symptoms of anxiety or even heart palpitations. Alcohol, when used long term, is known to decrease levels of serotonin; therefore, decreasing alcohol consumption will elevate serotonin levels, improving mood and decreasing anxiety and depression.

Supplements

Low levels of some B vitamins and folate (which is also a B vitamin with a different name) have been associated with depression and anxiety, as well as other mental health conditions. In fact, many patients who are treated with medications for such conditions do not improve until these vitamins are added to their regimen.[12] B vitamins and folate are involved in the production of the neurotransmitters serotonin, dopamine, and norepinephrine. The levels of these neurotransmitters affect a person's mood. Most commonly used antidepressant medications work to keep the levels in a normal range by inhibiting the breakdown of the neurotransmitters. However, if a person cannot produce enough of these neurotransmitters in the first place, the medications won't be as effective.

Botanical Therapy

Two well-known herbal preparations used in the treatment of anxiety are kava and valerian. Kava, originating in the western Pacific and found all over Polynesia, is traditionally served as a sedating drink. It is harvested from the roots of the plant and can be consumed as a standardized extract of purified kava lactones. The recommended dose is 50 to 70 mg three times per day. It can take four to six weeks to see an improvement. If the symptoms of anxiety are not sufficiently decreased, you could switch to valerian or a medication that your doctor prescribes.

Valerian can be found as a single remedy or as a component of a huge variety of teas, supplements, and tinctures. It is important not to combine

---

12. Richard C. Shelton, MD, et al., "Assessing Effects of l-Methylfolate in Depression Management: Results of a Real-World Patient Experience Trial," *Primary Care Companion for CNS Disorders* 15 (4): PCC.13m01520, doi:10.4088/PCC.13m01520.

sedating botanicals such as kava and valerian, either with each other or with sedating medications. Additionally, some people may experience a paradoxical effect from valerian, meaning that they may suffer more of a sense of excitation, stimulation, or insomnia. In fact, in the nineteenth century, valerian was used as a stimulant. The only way to know how valerian will affect you is to try it, so it would be best to initially keep the dose low, starting at 50 mg once a day and monitoring for side effects.

For depression, St. John's Wort may be effective. This flowering plant acts as a stimulant and is available in standardized doses of 300 mg, taken three times per day. It has been used for centuries, particularly in Europe, and is generally well tolerated.[13] It should not be taken with other antidepressants because St. John's Wort and modern antidepressants work in a similar way by making serotonin more available within the nervous system. Too much serotonin can lead to serotonin syndrome: symptoms include tremor, diarrhea, muscle stiffness, low body temperature, confusion, and possibly death. St. John's Wort can also weaken the effect of many commonly prescribed medications such as birth control pills, blood thinners, and heart medications. If you are planning to use St. John's Wort, you should discuss this with your health-care provider before starting.

Mind-Body Therapy

Various mind-body therapies can be used in the treatment of anxiety and depression, including meditation, yoga, guided imagery, tai chi, and qigong. These activities can calm the mind and relieve stress. It is best to choose one or two types of mind-body therapies that you enjoy and will perform regularly. Classes are increasingly available at community centers, gyms, and wellness centers. It is important to do your research to find a qualified teacher. There are many different styles within each

---

13. NIH National Center for Complementary and Integrative Health, "St. John's Wort for Depression: In Depth," https://nccih.nih.gov/health/stjohnswort/sjw-and -depression.htm, accessed June 30, 2017.

type of mind-body therapy, so you may have to try a few different classes until you find one that resonates.

Don't be afraid to shop around. Choosing the right practice, the right teacher, and the right venue is important. Some people may benefit from the social aspect of the class, but others prefer private instruction. All mind-body practices work well in combination with exercise, dietary changes, and botanical and pharmaceutical interventions, as well as in conjunction with psychotherapy, to decrease anxiety and stabilize mood. A nurturing mind-body practice can sustain you through a lifetime of emotional and physical challenges. With consistency, the benefits you receive will only deepen over time.

Acupuncture

Acupuncture, because of its ability to balance neurotransmitters, can be a useful adjunctive therapy in treating anxiety and depression. Severely depressed patients should not rely on acupuncture alone for relief of symptoms but may use acupuncture in combination with antidepressant medications and psychotherapy. For mild to moderate anxiety and depression, acupuncture can be an effective therapy even without medications. Acupuncture is particularly helpful in treating anxiety and depression in pregnant women because it avoids the use of medications that can cross the placenta and potentially harm the baby.[14]

Psychotherapy

An assessment by a psychologist or psychiatrist is certainly appropriate for anyone who suffers from anxiety or depression. This is especially true when symptoms are severe. Supportive psychotherapy can be combined with medications, lifestyle changes, and complementary therapies. There are many styles of psychotherapy, and it is important to be comfortable with both the therapist and the method.

---

14. David P. Sneizek, DC, MD, and Imran J. Siddiqui, MD, "Acupuncture for Treating Anxiety and Depression in Women: A Clinical Systematic Review," *Medical Acupuncture* 25 (3): 164–172, doi:10.1089/acu.2012.0900.

Pharmaceuticals

There are times when anti-anxiety and antidepressant drugs are warranted and even lifesaving. This class of drugs has a latency period, meaning that it may take several weeks to feel an improvement. If one drug of this type is not effective, then others can be tried instead, so it is important not to give up too soon. Once a suitable medication is found, the length of treatment can vary. Although the goal of any effective pharmacotherapy is to use the least medication for the shortest time, some people need to be on these medications for years in order to prevent relapses of severe, debilitating depression. If your doctor recommends these medications, it is important to take them as prescribed. Do not add supplements, decrease the drug dosage, or stop suddenly without discussing changes with your health-care provider.

Eastern Treatment Approach for Anxiety and Depression

Treating anxiety and depression with Eastern natural healing methods can be effective and have no side effects. Natural healing is whole-body healing, mind-body healing that involves many different methods and techniques. These methods can be used in combination, but they all work in harmony to create smooth energy flow in the body. As in Western medicine, Eastern medical practitioners recommend a healthy diet and balanced lifestyle but encourage additional modalities to help the patient achieve emotional stability and well-being as quickly as possible. These methods include Chinese herbal medicine, acupuncture, tui na (Chinese massage), tai chi, and qigong practice. Learning about the principles of Daoism and applying this philosophy to daily life can enhance the healing process. All these approaches aim to balance the body energy to restore equilibrium.

Natural healing involves the participation of the individual. It requires some work to make change. If we are not willing to do the work or not willing to make changes, we will likely remain dependent on conventional medicine and may have to deal with some of the side effects. Western medicine may offer quick relief of symptoms but may not address the root of the problem. Eastern healing methodology can offer long-lasting benefits, not only healing the current condition but also preventing future illness. Also, Eastern methodology may help to reduce the need for medication. With guidance from their medical providers and participation in their own healing, some people get off medication entirely.

Natural healing has always been central in Chinese culture. People consider that the foods they eat, the way they think, and the exercise and mental activities they perform all support a way of living that promotes physical and emotional well-being. Even in our modern world, many Chinese still keep this beautiful and balanced tradition, relying more on ancient practices than modern medicine for maintaining health, preventing disease, and treating illness, should it occur.

This sort of natural healing and health maintenance requires a multilayered approach. Learning and healing always go together, from theory to practice, so understanding the reasons for each activity prescribed is an important part of healing.

Understanding Yin and Yang

You may have heard the words "yin" and "yang," even before picking up this book. As we discussed in chapter 2, the concept of yin and yang is a Daoist principle that describes the universe as composed of pairs of opposites that balance and engender each other. This relationship is found everywhere, in everyday life, and in every kind of living system.

The theory of yin-yang is derived from age-old observations of nature and describes the way phenomena naturally group in pairs of opposites: heaven and earth, sun and moon, night and day, winter and summer, male and female, black and white, up and down, inside and outside, movement and stillness. These pairs of opposites are also complementary in that they depend on and counterbalance each other. Furthermore, they are mutually convertible, since either may change into its counterpart. The day eventually becomes night, and night eventually becomes day; a bad situation can become good, and good times can sour. In human life, as in all nature, nothing stays the same. Yin and yang are rooted in each other, and they are inseparable, interdependent, and mutually engendering. Without yin, there would be no yang. Without black, there would be no white (no contrast). Yin and yang counterbalance each other in the universe and within each person. Extreme yin can be weakening to yang and yang excess can be weakening to yin. The concept of yin-yang is found in everyday life, and it is at the core of the idea of energetic balance.

In disease and healing, understanding yin-yang theory is a big part of the practice of Eastern medicine. Using this notion of opposites, the patient can be brought back into balance. As practitioners of Eastern medicine, we help people regain their equilibrium.

For example, if an organ is weak, we use strengthening methods, and if the organ is in excess (overactive), we use reducing methods. If the person's qi is stagnant, we use dispersing methods to move the qi. If a patient's mind is racing uncontrollably, we use calming methods. These are some ways in which the theory of interdependent opposites is put into the practice of Eastern medicine.

Even in our daily lives, we can benefit from understanding the concept of yin and yang. For instance, if we work too much, we need a break so we can recharge our energy; if we eat too much, we can skip a meal or eat very lightly at the next meal; if we worry too much, think too much, or are stressed, we need to take time to meditate, to breathe, or to practice qigong and tai chi to allow our mind and body to meet and achieve balance. There is always a way. That is the Dao.

Be with the Dao

As we discussed earlier, Dao (sometimes written as "Tao") means the Way, following what is most natural, alive, and spontaneous. Its guiding principle is to follow what is natural to you so that your own inner nature will effortlessly unfold. So, everyone unfolds in different ways.

The only person you need to follow is yourself; you perform whatever is right for you. Many Buddhists, Christians, and Sufis study and practice the Dao because it helps ground the spirit into the body. The Daoist principles of qi, the life force, are in all creatures. They are based on balancing the receptive and expressive, or yin and yang, forces that resonate within everybody, every society, and every atom of nature. Thus, the original duality of being and nonbeing is mirrored in the dualities of the physical world. If one thing is difficult, there must be something else that is easy by comparison. The same is true for long and short, high and low, and so on. One of the keys to Daoist thought is the recognition of dualities. This is the yin and the yang.

All processes have active and passive principles. All physical conditions contain interdependent opposites, but many people think of these dualities as mutually exclusive. Instead of seeing active and passive parts of action as complements, we label one as good and make the other bad, and try to ignore or eliminate the "bad." Often, there is no absolute right and wrong; it depends on the situation. The more we understand this philosophy, the better we deal with our life stress.

The Dao is a beautiful path for everyday life and everyone who chooses to walk on it. It is simple, mild, smooth, soothing, pure, and still—yet it is also moving and present. It is in everything and has unbreakable power. The Dao is the way that has no end. We are learning the fundamental part of Daoist wisdom to help ourselves grow and restore long-term happiness.

The Dao teaches us to flow with nature but not against nature, to be plain and simple, to desire less and be satisfied with what we have, to walk on the path without analyzing the path, to be humble, to be gentle, to be easy, and to be simultaneously empty and full. This way we will be able to handle stress better at work and home, untangle our minds, and live peacefully.

Now, moving from theory to practice, we discuss specific Eastern modalities that can be used on your healing journey to achieve well-being in body, mind, and spirit.

Healing with Chinese Herbal Medicine

First, a word about safety. Herbs are drugs. Just as food has medicinal properties, so too do herbs. The majority of Western pharmaceuticals are derived from plants, so it should come as no surprise that herbs could have side effects if taken incorrectly or in conjunction with incompatible herbs, foods, or drugs. Purchasing herbal formulas off the internet or sharing someone else's herbs is highly discouraged. Before a practitioner of Eastern medicine prescribes an herbal formula, a lot of information is gathered from the patient to ensure optimal outcomes with minimal adverse effects.

Chinese herbs are used in various combinations, unlike Western herbs and medications, which are generally used individually. These herbal formulas are elegantly constructed, creating combinations that enhance the actions of each component and, at the same time, minimize possible side effects. In Chinese herbal prescriptions, different combinations of herbs influence the function of the organ-channel energy networks in the body.

In Eastern medicine, the organs are described as being associated with specific channels. These pairs of organs and channels create energy networks that have particular functions. Chinese herbal medicine is effective in balancing these energetic networks, harmonizing the body and the mind. In Western terms, this is akin to using pharmaceuticals to modulate organ physiology.

Herbal formulas can be cooked by the patient from raw herbs prescribed by the practitioner, reconstituted from granules and sipped as a tea, or taken in pill form. Pills or tablets are easier to take, but may not be as potent as cooked herbs or teas. Sometimes a patient is started on cooked herbs and then transitioned to pills for maintenance.

Regardless of the formulation, the most important aspect of herbal therapy is making the correct diagnosis within the paradigm of Eastern medicine. Only then can the correct formula be prescribed. For this reason, patients should consult a qualified professional herbalist who is trained in Eastern medicine. In Eastern healing, even though several people can have the same Western diagnosis, such as anxiety, depression, insomnia, or another ailment, the best herbal formula for each of those people may be different. Everyone has a different constitution. Some patients have an inherent vulnerability in one or more organ systems. In Eastern medicine this is referred to as a weakness or excess of organ energy.

Herbal formulas can be used in conjunction with other Eastern healing modalities such as acupuncture, tui na (Chinese massage), meditation, qigong, and tai chi. Also, appropriate dietary changes and exercise will help speed your recovery. Ideally, as your condition improves, your reliance on herbs may diminish. You may find that consistent attention to healthy food choices, persistent cultivation of your meditation, qigong and tai chi practice, and acupuncture or tui na as needed will help you maintain emotional and physical stability. At that point, you can consult with your Eastern practitioner about diminishing or discontinuing your herbal formula. Similarly, if you are taking Western medications, you can speak to your doctor about modifying your regimen.

Remember that everyone is different. Some people must take herbs or medications for a longer time than others, but incorporating all these recommended healing practices will increase the likelihood of long-lasting results.

Healing with Acupuncture and Tui Na (Chinese Massage)

Acupuncture is an effective treatment for a "tune-up" of the organ-channel system. It reduces the excesses, supports the weaknesses, and promotes a smooth flow of energy within the body. Tui na (Chinese deep massage) has similar effects. Tui na therapy can also be used in conjunction with herbs and acupuncture to unblock the stagnant qi and promote circulation. Both acupuncture and Chinese massage may involve multiple visits, depending on the severity of your symptoms. Either method can greatly enhance healing results if you combine acupuncture and tui na with tai chi or qigong practice.

Both modalities can be very effective when you find well-trained and experienced practitioners; however, if after several weeks of treatment you do not feel any improvement, we suggest that you return to your primary care provider for further evaluation. You may also choose to seek out another Eastern practitioner. Just as there are variations among Western practitioners, there are also differences in skill and expertise among Eastern practitioners. Do not deprive yourself of the healing aspects of acupuncture or tui na if your first treatments are not successful. Acupuncture and Chinese massage work very well for sufferers of mild and moderate depression and anxiety. For severe symptoms, you should be treated with both Eastern and Western medicine. Where you sit on the continuum of emotional well-being can shift quickly, so it is wise to involve both your Eastern and Western health-care providers.

Healing with Diet

A healthy diet can play an important role in preventing and healing depression and anxiety. As we discussed previously, a diet that is abundant in vegetables and healthy fats will decrease chronic inflammation in the body, which has been linked to depression as well as cardiovascular disease and diabetes.[15]

From years of experience, I (Dr. Kuhn) have found that predominantly plant-based diets and eating habits help balance the emotions. Therefore, I recommend that people try the following:

1. Eat a partial vegetarian diet. This means you eat less meat, more vegetables. Although you may think a complete vegetarian diet is healthier, you may not eat the variety of foods required for maximum nutrition. In addition, a completely vegetarian diet may not provide you with a feeling of fullness. Feeling satisfied after a meal can help prevent overeating. Some people who eat a vegetarian diet eat too much cheese or sweets, which can cause weight gain.

---

15. A. Sanchez-Villegas and M. A. Martinez-Gonzalez, "Diet, a New Target to Prevent Depression?" *BMC Medicine* 11 (3), http://biomedcentral.com/1741-7015/11/3.

2. Eat a variety of foods, including the foods you like and foods that may be less familiar. You should eat foods with all colors, all flavors, all textures, and all types of cooking styles. If you do so, you'll have a balanced diet, which can lead to balanced energy and emotions. This also provides a wider spectrum of nutrition to your body and helps the body maintain balanced organs. I have found that fussy eaters have more emotional issues than non-fussy eaters.

   A diet with a wide variety of foods is good for our digestive system. Our stomach releases certain enzymes when certain foods are ingested. If you are a fussy eater, your stomach may produce less of the enzymes needed to break down food groups that you do not eat. Then your body becomes sick when that specific food is introduced to the body, because it cannot be easily digested. I had a patient who was on a vegan diet and after a while she became anemic. Her doctor recommended that she eat red meat. She did what her doctor suggested, but she became very sick and her entire stomach malfunctioned. Her stomach could not produce the enzyme for red meat, and therefore her body reacted in a very negative way. She had pain, cramps, diarrhea and vomiting, and unintentionally lost a lot of weight.

3. Eat in moderation. Overeating is a big problem in many countries, particularly during the holiday season. We have a lot of fun at holiday parties, but we often feel bloated, tired, or even sick after we overeat. Overeating causes blockage in your digestive system, which, in Chinese medicine, includes the stomach and the spleen. These two organs are very important in maintaining energy levels and immune function. Low energy levels can make depression and anxiety worse. Emotional eating is another obstacle to healing. Long-term emotional eating does a lot of harm to our body and brain.

4. Eat natural foods and avoid processed foods. In the process of refining, foods lose nutrition, so they may be lacking in certain vitamins and minerals. Processed foods contain preservatives, which may prevent the foods from being completely digested,

absorbed, and used for energy. This not only makes the body gain weight or fat, but also makes the body vulnerable to stress; therefore, the emotions can be out of balance. If you eat more foods with preservatives, you may also have allergies or sensitivities, which can show up as skin problems, digestive problems, respiratory problems, or energy problems. When you have these problems, your mood can be disrupted.

5. Avoid eating late. Eating late contributes to weight problems, high blood pressure, high cholesterol, and insomnia. Two hours before bedtime you should only drink water. Do not eat food. You burn fewer calories at night and your circulation is slower at night. Therefore, we need fewer calories. Also, avoiding stimulants such as tea, coffee, and sugar can help you have restful sleep. Restorative sleep is essential to healing.

6. Drink more water. Some people live on soda, juice, and other sugary beverages, which can contribute to diabetes, heart disease, metabolic disease, and pain. Many people don't drink enough water because they either forget or dislike the taste.

   Water is the most important component in our body! Our body and our brain are mostly water. Water participates in every metabolic process in our body. You can live without food for three weeks but you would die without water in just three or four days.

   Water is needed by our brain to manufacture hormones and neurotransmitters; water regulates body temperature; water is needed by our stomach for enzymes to digest food; water allows body cells to grow; water forms saliva; water lubricates joints, maintains muscle mass, helps to detoxify the body, and accounts for a large portion of our blood volume.

   Although no optimal amount has been definitively determined, strive to drink about 64 ounces of water per day. Your activity and environment may dictate your needs. For example, if you do more physical work or live in a hot climate, you will need more water.

Dehydration occurs when you have lost 1 to 2 percent of your total water stores. Symptoms from dehydration include headache, dizziness, light-headedness, nausea, fatigue, shortness of breath, and mental fog. Try drinking more water every day to see whether your symptoms resolve.

7. Avoid using alcohol or drugs to even out your emotional ups and downs. Though alcohol is legal for adults, it can do a lot of harm. In Eastern medicine, the liver is associated with emotions, particularly anger. Alcohol can impair the physical functioning of the liver organ as well as the flow of liver energy. You may notice that someone who drinks excessively may have anger issues and relationship problems. This sort of self-medication may make you feel good at the time, but afterward, the essential issue that drove you to these substances is still there. Drinking alcohol or using drugs in this way is a temporary solution and does not get to the root of the problem. Unintended consequences such as accidental overdose and addiction are becoming more common in our society. Using natural healing methods to solve mental health concerns is much safer. If you feel you have a substance use disorder, it is imperative that you contact your primary care provider for help.

Healing with Tai Chi and Qigong

Tai chi and qigong are ancient methods of healing that incorporate movement, breath control, and meditation. Tai chi, also called *taijiquan* in Chinese culture, has been known for centuries for its health benefits, including mental benefits. Now, since the world has recognized its healing benefits, more and more people practice tai chi all over the world. Tai chi is a higher level of qi practice, or some say a "higher level qigong." Both tai chi and qigong are excellent methods for reducing anxiety, depression, and sleep difficulties. For beginners, starting with qigong is a good idea. For this reason, we focus on qigong and have devoted a whole chapter to this discussion (chapter 5). In the paragraphs that follow, we introduce some concepts about tai chi and qigong.

Practicing tai chi and qigong helps us stay in the present moment. When you are practicing tai chi, your mind is focused on learning and moving with controlled energy. Once you learn to stay in the present, you automatically detach from the "monkey mind." The term monkey mind is the label attached to your internal voice, the voice you hear in your mind that constantly chatters in the background as you go about your day.

Over time, by practicing tai chi or qigong, you will learn to be aware of the monkey mind but not to react to its narrative. You will feel calm, peaceful, centered, grounded (rooted). You may feel a smooth flow of the qi (energy); you may become more positive, stronger, and better able to face negatives situations with ease. You eventually will be able to shift your energy. Other benefits of practicing tai chi and qigong are improved digestion and metabolism, improved sexual functioning, increased blood circulation and cardiovascular fitness, increased youthfulness, and longevity.

Tai chi and qigong practice is a positive chain that consists of smoothing energy flow, letting go of negative thoughts, and becoming more positive and open to all. Both tai chi and qigong come from Daoist practice and involve balance and nature. All movements entail the yin and yang: constantly shifting weight and turning the waist; left and right, up and down, empty and full, stillness and movement, mind and body, breath in and breath out.

For anxiety and depression, a doctor will frequently prescribe medication such as antidepressants for at least one year to ensure long-term effectiveness. Many patients are not able to continue this treatment long-term and may discontinue their medication because they feel it's not working or because of the negative side effects. By starting to learn and practice tai chi or qigong, I (Dr. Kuhn) have found that the length of time patients need to take antidepressant medications can be reduced. I have also found that these practices help patients respond to their medication better, as well as reduce side effects of the drugs.

When a person has emotional issues, I feel that two things need to be addressed. First, your mind is troubled or your brain is not balanced. Second, your qi is stagnant or not flowing the way it is supposed to flow. Tai chi and qigong practice corrects these problems by using special body movements and patterns of breathing to focus the mind and promote the smooth flow of energy in the body. In the process, the energy between your mind and your body is also balanced. Tai chi and qigong redirect energy, promote circulation, strengthen muscles and joints, and uplift your emotions. The key is regular practice.

Because the movements involved in qigong are concise and simple to learn, we recommend developing a qigong practice first. For qigong exercises to help alleviate anxiety and depression, as well as insomnia, please see chapter 5.

Characteristics of Qigong

- It is easy to learn, easy to remember, and easy to practice.
- It empowers the mind, strengthens the body, and improves stamina and self-esteem.
- Its symmetrical movements balance both sides of the brain to harmonize brain activity.
- The movements involve learning that stimulates brain functions.
- The slow and balanced movements calm and balance the brain neurotransmitters, acting as a "natural tranquilizer."
- The gentle physical movement enhances energy flow in the body and improves daily energy levels.
- The localized steps require a small space to practice and can be practiced indoors when the weather is inclement.
- The coordinated, soothing movements improve coordination and balance, open energy channels, and help you open up to nature when practicing outdoors.
- Most movements are slow, soothing, calming, graceful, peaceful, and are especially suitable for the older generation and those with a chronic illness. Therefore, it is called the best healing exercise.

How Does Qigong Help with Depression and Anxiety?

1. Learning

   Learning is a big part of healing, especially in the healing of emotions. Our emotion center in our brain needs to be refreshed, nourished, stimulated, and balanced. When you start to learn things you are not familiar with, you start to shift your focus onto new knowledge, new approaches, and a new life. This sort of internal transformation can improve your situation in life. It is as if you are shifting negative energy to positive energy. The more positive energy you have, the better chance that you can be healed. Once you focus on learning qigong, and then start to practice diligently, your form will become more graceful and beautiful. This gives you a feeling of accomplishment and satisfaction. No matter how old you are, learning can always benefit your physical and emotional health.

2. Specific and balanced movements

   Qigong is very soothing and relaxing, and has open-framed movements that help open the energy channels. The movements are symmetrical, to harmonize both hemispheres of the brain. It is like a natural tranquilizer that immediately calms your mind and your body. The brain has two hemispheres, which carry out different functions. Most people have dominance of one side or the other in their brain function: some people are strong in language, whereas some people are strong in shape and space recognition, and time, but weak in communication. Some people learn certain things quickly and other things slowly. Generally speaking, men are stronger on the left side of their brain, woman are stronger on the right side of the brain. But some men are stronger on the right side and some women are stronger on the left side too. If you overuse the dominant side of the brain throughout your life, and fail to use the minor side of your brain, that side may lack stimulation and an imbalance can occur. Qigong exercise balances both sides of the brain, so you develop a well-balanced brain, improving cognitive skills, communication skills, social skills, and so on.

I had the chance to observe some of the greatest qigong masters from China. All of them are super smart, in all dimensions: social skill, logical thinking, intuition, and structured teaching. In addition, their physical stamina is incredibly strong and vibrant.

3. Create the smooth qi (energy) flow in the body

Qi is vital energy, or life force. It is the energy that underlies everything in the universe. Qi in the human body refers to the various types of bioenergy associated with human health and vitality. Qi controls the function of all parts of the body.

4. Group energy

For many centuries, human beings were always involved in group activities, functions, performances, and other social events. Human beings are social beings. Tai chi practice brings out a great deal of group energy and is most often practiced in group settings, either in a classroom or outdoors. This method of practice fosters discussion, friendship, and all the positive benefits of group energy. Because the energy of each individual affects the energy of others during practice, everyone feels good.

5. Martial art involvement

In qigong, some of the movements have some martial relevance. People choose to practice qigong for different reasons, such as to find inner peace, for healing, for martial art or self-defense, for relief of stress, for longevity, to maintain good health or for disease prevention, for flexibility, and for increasing energy and stamina. Qigong and martial arts predate tai chi. Compared with qigong, more of the movements in tai chi have a martial art aspect and can be used for self-defense. Those martial art movements found in qigong do make you feel stronger, especially internally.

Other Self-Healing Homework and Practice

1. Exercise regularly.

   Whether it is a Western or Eastern form, exercise is important. You can choose to do jogging, walking, running, swimming, tennis, a ball game, hiking, tai chi, qigong, martial arts, aerobic exercise, Zumba, yoga, whatever you enjoy.

2. Practice being positive.

   It is not easy to be positive all the time, but it can be done with practice. When you have a positive attitude, people like to be with you, they feel cheerful, and they feel good when you are around. Not many people like to be with someone who is negative or depressed. You lose friends that way. When you have no friends, depression becomes more pronounced. It is like a negative circle, everything becomes worse and worse. Without a change in attitude, or a change in the way of thinking, antidepressants are less likely to be helpful.

   I have seen many patients who heal at different rates. The main difference in their healing is their attitude; the way they think influences how they act. The one who is more positive heals faster than the one who is negative.

3. Avoid overanalyzing.

   There are major differences between Western psychology and Daoist healing. Western psychology tries to analyze everything, looking for reasons for everything. Sometimes, when you try so hard to find a reason, or try to find the exact answer, try to be so smart, you may create an ongoing battle within yourself. You may understand the cause of the problems, but may not know how to get rid of them.

   In Daoist healing and Daoist psychology, we practice letting go. Not everything is fair, not everything can be reasoned out, but everything does have a reason. Do we have to know everything?

No. When we are able to let go, we feel like we just unloaded five hundred pounds off our shoulders. This may not always be easy, but it can be done with mindful practice. When you are able to do that, your spirit and energy are lifted right away.

Some people worry about things that may never happen, which is a complete waste of energy. Cautiousness is good to have, in order to deal with situations that are unexpected. But being overcautious, worrying too much, and being always nervous creates negativities and blockages in the mind and loss of enjoyment of life.

People who think too much, worry too much, plan too much, and fear too much can create stress and tension, and then trigger depression, anxiety, and panic attacks.

We cannot control everything that can happen or that has happened in the past. We cannot predict everything that may happen in the future. We can only be prepared, try to manage our current situation within our ability, and live in the moment. Overanalyzing is a waste of our energy. It's better to preserve our energy for the important things we want to do: to strive for better health, happiness, and well-being. Then, when bad things happen, we will always find ways to deal with them.

4. Practice forgiveness.

> "True forgiveness includes total acceptance. And out of acceptance, wounds are healed and happiness is possible again."
>
> —Catherine Marshall (American author)

Forgiving is a very good practice for healing. Forgiveness creates positive energy and helps us to let go with ease. When we forgive, we feel free, open, happy, and relaxed. We all make some mistakes in our lives, and we all learn from mistakes. If we forgive, the love grows. Love can reinforce forgiveness and forgiveness can nurture love. They do go hand in hand. Hate is the opposite. It creates negative energy and it is an obstacle to healing.

5. Be with the Dao.

We have learned much about Dao. Now it is time to practice. Let's be more natural and spontaneous; let's be more relaxed, accepting, tolerant, appreciative, and positive.

Chinese people have used Daoism for centuries. In almost every field, people use Daoism to find the right answer for their own needs. Why don't we take advantage of this philosophy and use this ancient wisdom to help ourselves? This wisdom does not directly tell you what to do, but it does give you a light and direction to help you to see things more clearly. It teaches you to unload yourself, free your mind, and let things happen spontaneously and naturally. Overreacting to people or situations can cause conflict. If you stay focused, calm, and nonjudgmental, you can resolve many problems and overcome many "obstacles." If you go against the natural flow, you may worsen these "obstacles"; healing needs the natural flow.

With Daoist study and practice, you can be happy whether you are rich or poor, at any intellectual level or occupation, and at any age.

6. Be patient.

Healing takes time. Don't get discouraged or frustrated if you don't feel better immediately. Time allows you to learn, heal, find happiness, and achieve your goals. Be patient, but don't waste time; use it wisely to create the environment you need to nourish your spirit.

7. Focus on the present.

Staying focused on the present is a tough thing for many people. Our minds are always active and busy. We have so many distractions in our lives. It seem the busier we are, the more stress we have. We get preoccupied by pressing work deadlines, raising children, maintaining houses, paying bills, investing money, and planning for vacations and retirement. All these tasks are important and deserve attention, but often we try to do everything at once. We try to multitask. When we are doing more than one thing, our mind is in a different place. The commotion of the day can even appear in our dreams when we are sleeping!

In order to be productive and accomplish our work with less stress, we need to focus on the present; focus on whatever we are doing at this moment. This is mindfulness.

8. Good sleep helps healing.

No matter how stressful your day has been, do whatever you can to ensure a good night's sleep. In chapter 1, we discussed the connection between sleep and mental health. In the next chapter, we go into greater detail about normal and abnormal sleep patterns, external factors that influence sleep, and give you strategies for improving the quality and quantity of your sleep to restore energy and enhance healing.

The True Wellness Approach to Anxiety/Depression

- **Seek help from a qualified health-care provider to determine whether the seriousness of your condition warrants potentially lifesaving medications or counseling.**
- **Enjoy cardiovascular exercise most days of the week.**
- **Learn qigong or tai chi exercises.**
- **Meditate.**
- **Optimize the quality and quantity of your sleep.**
- **Increase your intake of omega-3 fatty acids (1–2 grams of EPA/ DHA daily), B vitamins, and folate (Vitamin B Complex plus 400 mcg of folate).**
- **Decrease your consumption of caffeine and alcohol.**
- **Consider kava, valerian, St. John's Wort, or Chinese herbal formulas as prescribed by a knowledgeable herbalist.**
- **Receive acupuncture treatments from an experienced practitioner.**
- **Maintain your social connections.**

CHAPTER 4

The True Wellness Approach to Sleep Disorders

WHAT CONSTITUTES A GOOD NIGHT'S SLEEP? Adequate quantity and quality of sleep such that you wake refreshed. Regarding the quantity of sleep, the number of hours you need depends on your age. According to the Centers for Disease Control, the amount of sleep recommended for adults age 18 to 60 is seven hours or more. Contrary to popular belief, older adults actually need about the same, between seven to nine hours per night. Teenagers need eight to ten hours and young children need even more than that![1] Unfortunately, for adults over the age of 18, at least one-third of us are averaging less than seven hours of sleep in a twenty-four-hour period.[2]

With respect to the quality of your sleep, this depends on many factors: Whether you have an underlying medical condition such as chronic pain, whether you take medications or supplements that alter your sleep stages and brain waves, whether you are naturally a light or heavy sleeper, whether you are a shift worker, and many more factors that we will discuss in the coming pages.

---

1. Centers for Disease Control, "How Much Sleep Do I Need?," https://www.cdc .gov/sleep/about_sleep/how_much_sleep.html (accessed March 12, 2019).

2. Centers for Disease Control, "Short Sleep Duration Among US Adults," https:// www.cdc.gov/sleep/data_statistics.html (accessed March 12, 2019).

In chapter 1, we discussed sleep in relation to emotional health and disease. We touched on some aspects of what happens in your brain when you sleep, but we have not yet described the full sleep cycle. Thanks to the scientists who have dedicated their lives to this area of study, we are learning more every year about the intricate biochemical and neurological dance that occurs during the different stages of sleep. It is well beyond the scope of this book to delve into the details of sleep physiology, so we will highlight important points to clear up common misconceptions about sleep. For those readers interested in a closer look at this fascinating subject, we recommend *Why We Sleep* by Dr. Matthew Walker.[3]

We would like to mention three essential pieces of information presented by Dr. Walker that may change the way you approach your sleep habits.

First, while your brain contains a natural timekeeper that keeps track of the twenty-four-hour circadian rhythms that govern your wakefulness, there is another mechanism that determines when you feel sleepy. Dr. Walker calls that mechanism "sleep pressure." This is how it works: From the time you wake, your brain is producing a chemical called adenosine. As the concentration of adenosine increases, you become increasingly sleepy. Peak concentrations occur between twelve to sixteen hours from the time you wake up. This would be around the time you would normally go to sleep. When you sleep, your adenosine levels drop. But, have you ever stayed up all night to finish a report or a school assignment and noticed that as you keep working into the early morning hours you get a "second wind?" Even though your adenosine levels continue to rise because you have not slept, your circadian rhythm that governs wakefulness is on the upswing. These two systems march along, quite independent from each other. Even though your wakefulness will wax and wane over a twenty-four-hour period, your adenosine levels will increase until you succumb to the pressure to sleep.[4] While caffeine can

---

3. Matthew Walker, PhD, *Why We Sleep: Unlocking the Power of Sleep and Dreams* (New York: Scribner, 2017).
4. Ibid., 36.

temporarily block the adenosine receptors, once the caffeine is out of your system, the even-higher levels of adenosine will activate the parts of your brain that initiate sleep. Therefore, it is best to pay attention to your feelings of sleepiness and minimize the use of caffeine.

Second, a full night's sleep is divided into approximately five ninety-minute cycles during which the various stages of sleep occur. These stages are divided into rapid eye movement sleep (REM) and non-rapid eye movement sleep (NREM). REM sleep is associated with dreaming and strengthening neural connections. NREM is further categorized as light and deep. Deep NREM sleep is the time during which the brain uncouples unimportant neural connections. Between these two mechanisms, your brain remodels and stores memories while you sleep. The crucial piece of information to understand is that the proportion of NREM to REM sleep changes over each of the five sleep cycles, with NREM sleep predominating early in the night and REM sleep accounting for the majority of the fifth cycle of the night. REM sleep is the most restorative. So, if you are sleeping for less than seven hours per night, you are missing out on the majority of your REM sleep that would occur in that fifth cycle.[5] People who wear devices that monitor their sleep may have noticed this phenomenon, that their deepest sleep is cut short by the need to wake up earlier than they would naturally.

Last, many people wake up for short periods of time between sleep cycles and then go back to sleep. So given what we have just learned about the different proportions of NREM to REM sleep during each cycle as we progress through the night, it is essential to give yourself the opportunity to sleep between seven and eight hours (five ninety-minute cycles). Therefore, you may need to give yourself a seven- to nine-hour window in which to realize what Dr. Walker calls this "sleep opportunity."[6]

There is a great deal more that Dr. Walker has to say about sleep, from the science of sleep to the societal implications of inadequate slumber. The problem is enormous. Sixty million Americans cannot sleep:

---

5. Ibid., 46.
6. Ibid., 261.

according to the National Institutes of Health, this is the number of people in this country who suffer from sleep problems every year. This may even be an underestimate, because these conditions frequently go undiagnosed. There are over eighty different types of sleep disorders. Many are extremely rare. It is not the purpose of this chapter to discuss each and every one of these ailments. We will touch on some of the most common sleep disorders, but will focus on insomnia. Aside from insomnia, some of the most common sleep problems include sleep apnea, narcolepsy, restless leg syndrome, and shift work disorder.

A person with sleep apnea will stop breathing multiple times during the night, sometimes as many as hundreds of times. This can be associated with heavy snoring, gasping, or choking. These periods of apnea (breathing stoppages) decrease the oxygen levels in the body and can lead to high blood pressure and heart disease as well as daytime fatigue and other chronic illnesses. There are two types of sleep apnea. The most common is obstructive sleep apnea where there is partial of total blockage of the nose or upper airway during sleep. Central sleep apnea is less common and occurs as a result of improper brain signaling. Essentially, the brain loses some of its ability to automatically regulate breathing.

Narcolepsy is a neurological problem. The brain's sleep-wake cycles are dysregulated. In Type 1 narcolepsy, the patient has a low level of hypocretin, a neurotransmitter that assists in modulating sleep-wake cycles. People with narcolepsy experience extreme daytime sleepiness, sometimes to the point that they fall asleep suddenly and at inappropriate times. Some people with narcolepsy may also experience a sudden decrease in muscle tone and control. This is called cataplexy and can occur when the person experiences extreme emotions. Sleep paralysis is another form of narcolepsy in which the person is awake but unable to move or speak. This terrifying condition can occur during the transition from sleep to wakefulness. The body normally does not move during REM sleep when a person is dreaming. Once REM sleep is over, the mechanism that prevents body movement is reversed. In sleep paralysis, the synchronization of this transition is off. Many people have an episode of sleep paralysis during their lives, but that does not mean they have narcolepsy.

Restless leg syndrome is very uncomfortable. Patients can have numbness, pain, or other disturbing sensations in their legs that cause a strong urge to keep them moving and therefore disrupt their sleep.

Many people in today's society work a non-traditional schedule. Unfortunately, this can play havoc with their sleep-wake cycles, leading to poor sleep, constant fatigue and impaired concentration, and an increased risk for accidents and chronic illnesses.

All of the above sleep disorders require an assessment from a neurologist, preferably one who has done the extra training needed to become a sleep specialist. While behavior modification may improve a patient's sleep slightly in these situations, sleep apnea, narcolepsy, and restless leg syndrome may only improve with prescription medications or devices (as in the case of obstructive sleep apnea). For those people who have shift work disorder, establishing and maintaining a strict sleep schedule with ample sleep opportunity is essential. Behavioral changes, as we will discuss in reference to insomnia disorders, can also help normalize sleep for shift workers, but a change of employment may need to be considered in order to prevent serious health complications.

Insomnia disorder is generally defined as difficulty initiating or maintaining restorative sleep for at least four weeks, coupled with excessive fatigue or somnolence that results in impairment of daily functioning. Chronic insomnia is defined as insomnia that occurs at least three times per week for a minimum of three months. The categorization of insomnia is further broken down into primary and secondary insomnia. Primary insomnia is not caused by other medical or psychiatric illnesses. Secondary insomnia is a symptom of another disorder. Secondary insomnia will resolve when the initiating disorder is successfully treated. Insomnia, whether primary or secondary, is often left inadequately treated. Aside from the misery of being unable to sleep, insomniacs are at increased risk for subsequent serious medical conditions (known as comorbidities), including heart disease, cancer, diabetes, obesity, chronic pain, and neurological and digestive disorders. Persistent insomnia can also result in clinical depression, substance abuse disorders, anxiety disorders, increased risk of accidents, and decreased productivity.

The economic effect of insomnia has been estimated as high as $107 billion annually. Of this, almost $14 billion can be attributed to direct medical costs. Those who suffer from insomnia tend to utilize the healthcare system at a greater rate than those who sleep well. The enormity of the personal, societal, and fiscal burden of insomnia underscores how important sleep is to our overall well-being.

Insomnia can be an isolated ailment (primary) or associated with another disease (secondary). But it gets even trickier than that. Insomnia can be both the cause and the result of another condition. This is the classic "chicken or egg" conundrum. Which came first? Illness or insomnia? Did the sleep disorder predate or follow the onset of the comorbid affliction? Because of its complexity, the treatment of insomnia first requires a comprehensive assessment of the patient, looking for "predisposing, precipitating, and perpetuating factors" that can influence the disorder.[7] This is true in both Western and Eastern medical disciplines.

Predisposing factors include biomedical, psychological, and lifestyle influences. Biomedical illnesses that can predispose someone to insomnia include conditions that cause pain and prevent sleep, obstructive sleep apnea, and heartburn (gastroesophageal reflux). Psychological predisposing influences include clinical depression and anxiety. Lifestyle factors that can predispose a patient toward a sleep disorder are many, including excessive use of alcohol, caffeine, cigarettes, or illegal drugs; use of medications that alter the sleep/wake cycle; and occupational sleep disruptions such as rotating shift work, night work, and jet lag.

Stress is usually the precipitating factor that causes insomnia in predisposed individuals. It need not be a negative event that has triggered a person's inability to sleep. Positive, even joyful events, such as an

---

7. Rubin Naiman, PhD, "Insomnia," in *Integrative Medicine*, 4th ed., edited by David Rakel, MD, 74, (Philadelphia: Saunders/Elsevier, 2018).

upcoming marriage, job promotion, or purchase of a new home can cause persistent sleeplessness.

Finally, perpetuating factors include tactics that many people try in an effort to sleep. These include napping during the day, staying in bed even when not sleepy, and the long-term use of prescription sleep aids. Unfortunately, all these behaviors tend to make insomnia worse rather than better, particularly the use of sleeping pills. These addictive medications disrupt the normal phases of the sleep cycle, leading to non-restorative sleep and ever-increasing fatigue.

A wide variety of medications can not only cause insomnia but may also complicate its treatment, whether by Western or Eastern practices. A partial list of commonly used medications follows.

Medications that May Cause Sleep Difficulties

Blood pressure medication
> atenolol, metoprolol, propranolol
> clonidine
> hydrochlorothiazide
> losartan, valsartan, irbesartan

Heart arrhythmia medication
> procainamide, quinidine, disopyramide

Asthma medication
> theophylline, albuterol

Steroids
> prednisone, cortisone

Antidepressants
> fluoxetine (Prozac™), sertraline (Zoloft™)

Cholinesterase inhibitors (used in the treatment of neurological conditions)
> donepezil (Aricept™), galantamine (Razadyne™), rivastigmine (Exelon™)

Cholesterol reducing medications (statins)
    atorvastatin (Lipitor™), simvastatin (Zocor™), lovastatin (Mevacor™)

Thyroid medication
    levothyroxine

Smoking-cessation aids
    Nicoderm™, Nicorette™

Headache medication (contains caffeine)
    Excedrin™, Anacin™

Attention deficit disorder medication
    methylphenidate (Ritalin™), methamphetamine (Desoxyn™)

Western Pathophysiology of Insomnia

Recently, Western medicine has come to look on the disorder of insomnia as a state of "hyperarousal." Comparing people with insomnia to those without, insomniacs tend to have higher heart rates, elevated core body temperatures, increased body and brain metabolic rates, and amplification of specific types of brain activity. They also exhibit neuroendocrine disruption, as evidenced by abnormally high nighttime cortisol levels and decreased serum melatonin (the hormone that makes you sleepy). These and many other hormones are regulated by the hypothalamic-pituitary-adrenal axis. This is how your brain and adrenal glands talk to each other. When this system is overactive, as in the case of insomniacs, the adrenal glands create too many stress hormones. This, in turn, leads to chronic inflammation.

Such inflammatory conditions are often accompanied by anxiety, depression, and pain, leading to abnormal sleep patterns. In turn, even a single night of disturbed sleep can change the way your immune system functions and result in increased inflammation. This can lead to more pain and emotional distress, which further disrupts your sleep. If ever there were a vicious cycle, this is certainly it!

One would think that prolonged insomnia would result in sleepiness, but this is generally not the case. Unfortunately, insomniacs find themselves fatigued—but *not* sleepy. They are exhausted but hyperalert. This is in keeping with the state of hyperarousal that is associated with insomnia.

Insomnia includes many different subtypes; this is why it is important to speak to your doctor rather than try to manage this condition on your own. Different sleep disorders have different symptoms. You may have difficulty falling asleep or staying asleep for a variety of reasons. Such reasons could include a dysregulation of your "internal clock" (the part of your brain that controls your bodily functions and cycles), abnormally elevated nighttime body temperature, and difficulty breathing while asleep (known as sleep apnea). Concomitant illnesses, including psychiatric disorders, should be identified and addressed. For women, insomnia related to menstruation or menopause is not uncommon and can be treated. If your inability to sleep does not resolve by optimizing coexisting medical conditions, further action is warranted. Your doctor may refer you to a specialist who can conduct sleep studies to determine the cause of your insomnia. These days, sleep studies can be performed either in sleep labs or in your own home.

Western Treatment of Insomnia

Successful treatment of insomnia is predicated on proper nutrition, adequate exercise, and effective stress management. Of course, this could be said of almost any chronic degenerative condition. The management of insomnia, specifically, can be approached in two ways. The first method, the one that most people try initially, is taking something to help them sleep. The "something" can range from warm milk to herbal teas to alcohol to sleeping pills. Many people also consume botanical remedies or nutritional supplements in the hope of getting a good night's sleep.

Some of these remedies can be quite effective. Sufficient evidence supports the use of hops, valerian root, and melatonin as sleep aids; these should be used separately, rather than combined.

Hops are the flower clusters of the hop vine, used for making beer. Hops decrease muscle spasms and promote relaxation. Valerian root is a botanical that has long been used to decrease anxiety and increase feelings of tranquility.

Melatonin is the hormone that your brain secretes to promote sleep. During the day, exposure to the blue wavelength of light inhibits the production of melatonin, allowing you to stay awake. When night falls, the lack of blue wavelength light permits the brain to manufacture more melatonin. Ironically, by staying up late, using artificial light sources, and watching television or using computers, we are bathing ourselves in blue wavelength light at an inappropriate time of day. As a consequence, we are inadvertently interfering with our ability to produce melatonin. This hormone is also known to have anti-inflammatory, antioxidant, and anticancer properties. It is thought that the suppression of melatonin may contribute to the expression of many medical conditions, not just insomnia.

Hops, valerian root, and melatonin have excellent safety profiles, though in some people, valerian acts as a stimulant rather than a sedative, as we mentioned in the previous chapter. Overall, hops, valerian, and melatonin are non-addictive and do not interfere with brain functions such as memory consolidation and problem solving. (Specific dosing and recommendations for these remedies can be found at the end of this chapter.)

In contrast, medications commonly used to promote sleep fail to replicate normal sleep patterns, thus interfering with the brain's ability to recall memories and function correctly. Long-term use of prescription sleep aids is not recommended and can result in amnesia, cognitive impairment, rebound insomnia, dependence on ever-increasing dosages of hypnotic medication, and even death.

The prime directive of Western medicine is "do no harm." The common practice of repeatedly renewing prescriptions for sleeping pills is in direct violation of this principle. This is why, if you are a chronic insomniac, you should be referred to specialists who are trained to root out the underlying cause of your persistent sleeplessness. Such an endeavor takes time—something a general practitioner may not have in great quantities. Sleep specialists also look at insomnia from a different point of view than most patients and many doctors. The majority of people look at insomnia as a lack of sleepiness, but, in keeping with the hyperarousal model, sleep specialists characterize most types of insomnia as "excessive wakefulness."

The first method of treating insomnia caused by a lack of sleepiness is to "take something," such as hops or melatonin, as we discussed. However, if you are excessively alert, the second method of treating insomnia should be employed. This requires you to "give something up." In this case, the "something" to give up is the constant tension and chatter that is percolating through your body and mind, along with decreasing the disturbances within your sleep environment. This method of treatment, developed by leading integrative medicine sleep specialist Dr. Rubin Naiman, is called the noise-reduction approach to insomnia (NRAI).[8]

This approach conceptualizes "noise" as all the biomedical, psychological, and environmental factors that contribute to the abnormal hyperalert state. Using this framework, "body noise," "mind noise," and "bed noise" can be identified and systematically reduced.

Body Noise

To decrease body noise, comorbid medical conditions and lifestyle choices must be addressed and the cause of insomnia "given up." For example, if you have back pain that is keeping you awake, your doctor should investigate the cause and refer you for proper treatment to alleviate the pain. It is obvious that you will sleep better if you are not in pain, but the reverse is also true. It has been shown that deep sleep can increase your pain tolerance by 60 to 200 percent. If some of your medications have insomnia as a prominent side effect, perhaps your doctor can switch you to an alternate medication that will achieve the desired goal without disrupting your sleep. If you drink seven cups of coffee each

---

8. Ibid., 80.

day, you need to start weaning yourself until you reach an acceptable maximum of about three cups per day.

Mind Noise

The emphasis in the process of mind noise reduction is tackling the psychological and behavioral maladaptations that are keeping you awake. This involves taking a close look at your sleep habits and your beliefs about sleep, stress, and dreams.

More often than not, insomniacs lie in bed in a state of alertness. Their muscles are tense and may even ache. They often describe an inability to "turn off" their minds. Many insomniacs can't stop thinking. They are ruminating about the events of the day or things that happened in the distant past. They often worry about what may happen in the future. Above all, they are fretting about how much they really need to go to sleep! Because of these mental and emotional features of insomnia, cognitive-behavioral therapy has become one of the first line treatment recommendations made by sleep specialists.[9] Cognitive-behavioral therapy for insomnia, known as CBT-I, addresses the beliefs people hold about sleep that causes excessive anxiety and dysfunctional thoughts about their sleep performance. Many people set themselves up for frustration and disappointment if they think they must fall asleep quickly, sleep deeply through the night without waking at all, and accomplish all this by sheer force of will. Cognitive-behavioral therapy for insomnia helps people to set realistic expectations about sleep and develop habits that promote the transition from wakefulness to sleep. These habits are commonly known as "sleep hygiene." Proper sleep hygiene alone will not cure prolonged insomnia, but these beneficial habits are an effective component of a multifaceted treatment strategy that includes cognitive-behavioral therapy. Studies have shown that CBT-I is at least as effective as prescription sleep aids in the treatment of insomnia. The positive effects of CBT-I were long-lasting and without major side effects.[10]

---

9. Ibid., 74.
10. Ibid., 81.

During CBT-I, patients are asked to reconsider the beliefs that provoke anxiety about sleep, or rather, the lack of it. Probably the most difficult belief for people to give up is the idea that they should stay in bed until they fall asleep. This is extremely counterproductive. You cannot make yourself fall asleep. Sleep is not under your conscious control. Lying in bed and hoping desperately to fall asleep will only increase your anxiety. Increased anxiety leads to increased alertness. Increased alertness tells your primitive brain that you could be in danger. Stress hormones are then released in preparation for a possible fight or flight. An animal wouldn't fall asleep if it sensed danger, and neither will you.

So, how to call a halt to this unhealthy spiral? Get out of bed. This is the essence of a treatment called "stimulus control therapy." It is used to redirect behavioral responses to insomnia so you don't end up making the situation worse. Stimulus control therapy is used in combination with other treatment approaches and should *only* be used while being supervised by a sleep specialist. This method is contraindicated in patients who have sleep apnea, bipolar disorder, or epilepsy, or who are at risk for falling or have parasomnias; parasomnias include sleepwalking, sleeptalking, night terrors, and deep-sleep (rapid eye movement, or REM) disorders. If you suffer from any of the above illnesses, you should *not* try stimulus control therapy.

However, if your insomnia is caused by another condition and has simply perpetuated itself, you could consider this approach if you are supervised by a sleep specialist. The steps are as follows:

- Use the bedroom only for sleep and sexual activity.
- Lie down to sleep only when you are actually sleepy.
- If you are awake after about fifteen minutes, get up and leave the bedroom. Do *not* turn on your television, computer, iPad, cell phone, or video games. Instead, perform a relaxing activity until you are sleepy.
- Go back to bed. If you haven't fallen asleep within about fifteen minutes or you start to feel anxious about sleeping, get up again.
- Repeat the process as needed until you fall asleep.

- Go to bed each night and wake up at the same time every morning regardless of how long you actually slept.
- Do not nap during the day until your sleep cycle has normalized.

Relaxation practices are essential to the success of this therapy but are also very important for the reduction of mind noise, even if stimulus control therapy is not used. The purpose of relaxation practices is to balance your central nervous system and decrease the sympathetic tone that is responsible for the fight-or-flight response. High levels of activity of the sympathetic nervous system will increase your state of alertness. The paired but opposite entity that balances the sympathetic nervous system is the parasympathetic nervous system. The parasympathetic nervous system is responsible for decreasing your heart rate and blood pressure, among many other functions. Relaxation practices bolster the parasympathetic nervous system and will help you reach the calm, tranquil state that is necessary to transition into sleep. Many, many techniques can be used to induce relaxation, including, but not limited to, the following:

- Breathing exercises
- Qigong and tai chi
- Yoga
- Meditation
- Biofeedback
- Self-hypnosis
- Guided imagery

It is important to find an activity that you find both relaxing and enjoyable. Readers who claim they find using electronic media relaxing and enjoyable are reminded that such practices increase activity within the sympathetic nervous system and decrease melatonin production because of blue wavelength light exposure. It is far better to use the qigong exercises presented later in this chapter for insomnia.

Another aspect in the reduction of mind noise is the restoration of "dream health." Although this may not be a characteristic interest of conventional Western medicine, more and more practitioners are recognizing the importance of dreams. Dreams occur during the phase of sleep called the rapid eye movement (REM) stage, which is integral to the processing of memory and emotion. Many medications interfere with this stage of sleep and consequently disrupt dreaming. Traumatic events and emotional stress can result in recurring dreams or nightmares, resulting in a fear of sleep, which can contribute significantly to insomnia. Discussing disturbing dreams with your health-care practitioner may help you determine the actions you need to take to reduce your stress and improve your health. It is interesting to note that an assessment of a patient's dream health has always been a part of Chinese medicine.

Bed Noise

Bed noise refers to the environment of your bedroom. This includes not just the physical space, but what goes on in it. Your bedroom should be a safe haven. It should be stress-free.

Sit on your bed and take a close look at your sleep environment. Are there electronics in evidence? If so, remove all of them: televisions, computers, cell phones, and games. Even move your clock so it is not a distraction at bedtime. Do you take work to bed, literally? Are there piles of reports to read or bills to pay on your nightstand? Find a new room for all work- or school-related items. Take a deep breath. How does your bedroom smell? Is it moldy, or do you notice any chemical smells that are evidence of outgassing from furniture, floors, or mattresses? Some people are very sensitive to synthetic materials that can make a bedroom toxic and cause insomnia. Any mold should be removed, by whatever means necessary. If you have chemical sensitivities, replace the offending items with natural products. Use a high-efficiency particulate air (HEPA) filter to improve the air quality in your bedroom.

Next, make sure your bedroom is truly dark at night. Is there a big fluorescent sign or street lamp that shines through your bedroom window? Make an investment in blackout curtains to ensure these outside light sources do not disrupt your body's ability to manufacture melatonin. Give your body a little extra help by dimming your house lights an hour or two before bedtime and using special blue wavelength blocking filters on your electronics. Both these tactics will encourage your brain to create sufficient melatonin.

Last, pause and ask yourself how you feel. Do you feel safe in your own bedroom? This refers to both physical and emotional security. Determine what needs to be done to restore tranquility to your bedroom. You may require the help of your doctor for deep-seated problems.

By using the noise-reduction approach to insomnia, in conjunction with modalities that your Western and Eastern practitioners may recommend, you will enhance the quality of your sleep and, subsequently, your health. For more information about Dr. Naiman's Noise Reduction Approach to Insomnia (NRAI), you can go to his website listed in our recommended reading and resources section.

You may want to use the following questionnaire to help pinpoint areas of your sleep routine that need attention. This self-assessment tool can also be used to monitor your progress as you institute your new sleep regimen. If your sleep quality and quantity is not improving even after making the suggested changes, please take your self-assessments to your primary care provider for further evaluation.

Sleep Hygiene Self-Assessment

Day:

Caffeine	No _____	Yes _____	How Much? _____
Nicotine	No _____	Yes _____	How Much? _____
Stimulants	No _____	Yes _____	How Much? _____
Alcohol	No _____	Yes _____	How Much? _____
Exercise	No _____	Yes _____	How Much? _____
Meditative practice	No _____	Yes _____	How Much? _____

Night:

Electronics turned off at least 90 minutes before
bedtime   No_____ Yes_____

Bedroom safe and cool   No_____ Yes_____

Use of sleep aids:

    Botanical/Supplements   No_____ Yes_____ Type?_____

    Prescription   No_____ Yes_____ Type?_____

Time to bed _____

Time to rise _____

Sleep Opportunity (hours between time to bed and time to rise)_____

Time awake during night _____

Hours of sleep (sleep opportunity – time awake during night)_____

Quality of sleep   Fitful _____ Restful_____

Energy level on waking (on a scale of 1–10/10, with 10/10
being highest)_____

Summary of Western Interventions for Insomnia

- Seek medical attention to specifically address your insomnia, requesting an evaluation of comorbid conditions that may disrupt your sleep.
- Minimize the use of alcohol, caffeine, nicotine, and other stimulants.
- Perform relaxation exercises daily.
- Assess bedroom for electronics, stressors, environmental toxicity, and personal safety.
- Use blue wavelength light filters on computer and television screens to improve your brain's melatonin production.
- Dim lights an hour or two before bedtime, and ensure exposure to light in the morning to help the body maintain a normal sleep/wake cycle.
- Consider the use of ONE of the following:

Melatonin: 0.3–0.5 mg before bedtime, with your doctor's approval.

Valerian: 300–900 mg standardized extract of 0.8 percent valerenic acid 30 to 120 minutes before bed. It may take several weeks of valerian use to determine its effectiveness.

Hops: 0.5–1 dropper full of five to one ethanolic extract, 30 to 60 minutes before bed.

- Ask your doctor for a referral to a sleep specialist if your insomnia persists.

Eastern Treatment Approach to Insomnia

Having a good night's sleep is so important. Most healing processes happen at night when the body/mind is completely at ease and relaxed. I (Dr. Kuhn) have seen many patients throughout my career and have asked every one of them whether they had good night's sleep. The ones who said "yes" healed faster; the ones who said "no" healed much more slowly. I then changed my strategy and treated their insomnia at the same time I addressed their other problems. The results were much better after I regulated their sleep, and their primary problem healed a lot faster.

There are many natural ways to deal with insomnia. But first, we need to identify the cause or causes. This is the underlying principle of the Eastern healing system. Without removing the causes, the insomnia can come back after a while. No matter what methods you use to help the insomnia, if you do not solve the underlying problem, the solutions remain superficial or provide only temporary relief.

As in the Western approach to insomnia, if your sleep difficulties are caused by medication that you use for other illness, you may need to think about how to use natural ways to help reduce the need for medication. In some cases, you may have to use medication for the rest of your life, but not in all cases. Who wants to use medication for a lifetime, anyway? If you want to reduce the amount of medication you are taking, you need to do everything you can to correct the underlying problem. For example, if your blood pressure medication is disturbing your sleep, get serious about changing your diet, exercising, meditating, and practicing qigong in order to decrease your need for that medication. You may surprise yourself and be able to get off medication completely.

Be sure to discuss medication changes with the prescribing physician before you decrease your dose. Many drugs have serious side effects if they are stopped suddenly. The dose must be reduced gradually. Qigong exercise and changing your diet is a very good way to improve your sleep while you are tapering your medications under supervision.

If your insomnia is caused by relationships, you may need to find ways to improve those relationships, or let go if the situation cannot be changed. No matter what, you will need to do something, otherwise you will need to use medication to help you sleep, and deal with the side effects of medication.

If your insomnia is caused by stress, find an effective way to reduce your stress. I had a patient some years ago who had severe insomnia. I asked her whether there was anything troubling her mind. She said she was worried about money because she had two houses and two mortgages to pay. I ask her what would happen if she sold one house and kept just one house. She said she wanted to have two houses. OK, then, she will have worry, insomnia, and consequently some other illness. Human desire is endless, never having enough. If you sit back and think a moment, what is important in life? Would health and happiness come from multiple houses, fancy cars, and a million dollars in the bank? Not really. I used to have two houses. But the endless housework gave me back pain; it was too much work! The pressure of paying too much in mortgage payments is not wise. I could have had more savings if I had learned to live more simply at that time. I am now living more simply and have created a stress-free life: no need to worry. I am happier; I have enough for food, a house, travel, taxes, and bills. Now I can relax.

Many people overthink their problems, making circles in their minds. Overthinking can create problems. This is inefficient and does not often lead to solutions; it has no end and can keep you up all night. I have seen so many people overthinking. They had anxiety, insomnia, depression, low energy, and poor immune function. An overused mind doesn't work efficiently. I often teach my patients to write everything down on a piece of paper to relax the mind. This way, you use your eyes instead of your mind. This method helps you make things happen by accomplishing each item on the paper, rather than overusing the mind, going in circles. Sometimes allowing your mind to run in circles can lead you to make wrong decisions. You will need to break this cycle by practicing meditation, qigong, tai chi, or yoga, whichever practice best calms your mind.

If your insomnia is caused by pain, dealing with the pain should be the first step. For example, if you have a neck problem, you can go to a medical professional or holistic medical professional to get help. In my training program "Wellness Tui Na Therapy," level II is "Back and Neck Therapy." This special therapy can help insomnia, headaches, dizziness, and other issues that Western medicine has difficulty treating. As the pain levels drop, sleep improves.

If your insomnia is caused by overexcitement, either positive or negative, you should immediately use appropriate techniques to keep your body and mind calm and even and restore inner peace. The techniques can be qigong, tai chi, yoga, meditation, stretching, deep breathing, whichever you feel is right for you. In my own experience, practicing qigong, even for just a few minutes, can help me to calm my mind and body.

If your insomnia is caused by a hormone imbalance, regulating hormones can help you sleep. In Chinese medicine, hormone imbalance indicates organ system imbalance. With appropriate herbal medicine, acupuncture, or qigong, hormones can be regulated naturally.

In some cases, insomnia is caused from eating at night. Generally speaking, you should not eat any high-calorie food or drink after dinner. Unfortunately, many people enjoy some snacks, junk food, or dessert after dinner, which can cause insomnia or a weight problem. Discovering and addressing the underlying reason that some people overeat at night can solve many sleep problems.

Regarding using sleeping pills, I had a patient who told me that she had the opposite reaction—they kept her awake all night. Most people can fall asleep using a sleeping pill. Unfortunately, the quality of sleep that results from the use of sleeping pills is not normal. Also, using sleeping pills over a long period of time not only causes more problems from side effects (discussed previously), but also they becomes less effective or addictive. If you have to use them under extreme circumstances, I recommend only occasional use. Everyday use is not recommended. Unfortunately, many people fear that they may be worse if they don't take the sleeping pill. You may feel tired if you don't get a good night's sleep, but once sleep is caught up on the next night, you will feel better the following day. Fear and anxiety around the inability to sleep can make your insomnia worse. It is best to avoid the use of sleeping pills altogether.

No matter what caused your insomnia, learning and practicing qigong and tai chi can help regulate your sleep. Tai chi and qigong are moving meditation. These slow exercises incorporate breath, mind, and body to help balance the autonomic nervous system, especially increasing vagus nerve function (parasympathetic nervous function). The vagus nerve regulates heart rate, breathing, blood pressure, and all other organ functions; when regulated, it is the key component of the central nervous system that improves sleep.

Natural Strategies for Insomnia

Many natural methods can successfully improve insomnia. If your insomnia is severe or chronic, you should seek medical help in addition to trying these useful tips. However, these tips are the beginning of a new sleep routine. It is not just a one-time practice or one-week practice. It may need to be a lifelong practice in order to maintain a disease-free life. It may be a life-changing experience. Once you instill the healthy habit, you will soon realize that everything starts to work together in your body.

1. Go to bed at the same time each night. Your body has a natural time reader and can read your pattern. If you have a regular pattern, your

body and the chemicals in the body work with you, not against you. If you don't have a regular pattern, your body can be confused, as in jet lag, which many of us have experienced. Or we can say our body works better with consistency. If you work the night shift, it is better to work the night shift regularly. I used to be an OB/GYN in China. The thing I hated most was that all doctors took turns doing night shift for one day or two, and then day shift for the next one or two days, which upset my sleeping pattern. I feel like I still have some of the lingering effect: sometimes I don't sleep well. Luckily, it is not all the time. Again, developing the discipline to keep a regular bedtime can help build a healthy habit and improve your sleep.

2. Do not eat or drink anything after dinner, except water. Many people don't do much after dinner, so the calories stay in their bodies and are slowly metabolized. In contrast, during the day-time your calories burn a lot faster from various work or exercise. After dinner you should not be hungry unless you go to sleep late. Most foods that we snack on at night are high in calories; we don't need more calories before we go to bed. If you go to sleep late, which I don't recommend, you can eat a celery stick or a carrot stick with nothing on it or some nuts if you are hungry.

3. Avoid watching an exciting movie at night. You can watch some-thing very light or humorous, but don't let anything get your emotions going or feeling upset or excited. I find it is very helpful to watch nature documentaries; after one or two episodes, I am ready to fall asleep. Such documentaries are usually very calming, with relaxing narration and music. My mind is relaxed; at the same time, I learn something, but not to the level of excitement. I feel very peaceful and at ease. At night, ease is important. Watching this kind of documentary film also takes your mind away from overthinking.

4. Stop thinking! I say this so often to my patients and to my students—some of them just think way too much. Overthinking is totally useless. It seems rude to say this, but what I really mean is to advise them to stop overthinking. We all think too much

sometimes. Our mind very often causes more problems and creates negative results. If we think just right, our mind helps us produce positive results. How do you think just right? Imagine a regular day: when it is time to work, we work; when it is time to go home, we go home. In our mind, it should be the same way: when it is time to think, we think; when it is time to rest, we rest. We learn to focus on whatever we are doing at this moment without worrying about the next moment. When the next moment comes, we focus on it. If we need to plan, we make some plans and write them down. At night, all we need is to relax our mind, to chill, to enjoy pleasant conversation, and to read either for learning or for leisure. If we do the opposite, we overthink or worry before we go to bed, and this most likely leads to insomnia. The next day we cannot think clearly, therefore it is counterproductive. After a while, our brain becomes foggy, our memory declines, we feel tired, and eventually we go to a doctor who most likely gives us the name of a disease—then, we are labeled.

5. Practice meditation. Practicing meditation is very beneficial to our body, mind, and brain. Meditation makes us more mindful, more focused, more alert, better in control of our emotions, and brings us to a higher level of well-being. Physically, it reduces blood pressure and heart rate, promotes digestion and absorption, and guides us to do the right things for our body such as exercise, eat well, and be a positive person.

You can meditate anytime and anywhere during the day. It can be five minutes, ten minutes, or twenty minutes, depending on how much time you have. Even a ten-minute meditation break during work can be beneficial—like taking a mini-vacation. All you need to do is make time to do it. Again, I am saying the same thing: no matter how much you know, it is not useful without practice. Some people say you have to meditate thirty to forty-five minutes to get results. This can be intimidating for busy people; they won't do it, because they don't have forty-five minutes. You can take less time to meditate, but do it more often and do it correctly; you can still get the benefits. It is better than not doing it at all. If you have never practiced meditation, here are some methods for you to try.

Position: Your body position should be very comfortable, either standing or sitting, or even lying on the ground, whatever feels most comfortable. If you prefer to sit on the floor, you may need a cushion or pillow to help your posture so that you won't have backache during meditation. If you choose to lie on the floor, you may fall asleep during meditation practice. This is because meditation makes you very comfortable and relaxed.

Mind: During meditation practice, you need to remove any thought in your mind. No matter how much work you have to do, you are not doing work but having a mini-vacation at this moment. You can do the work later.

First, your mind should focus on your breathing: how deep, how slow, how even. In the beginning, your breath may be too fast, but as you continue your daily practice, your will realize that you can breathe more deeply, more slowly, and with more intention.

Next, you need to focus on total relaxation. Ask yourself some questions: Are my shoulders relaxed? Is my neck relaxed? Is my back relaxed? Is my body comfortable? Make sure your answer to each is yes. If not, relax each part of the body at each exhalation until all parts of the body are relaxed.

You are meditating now; it is not the right time for you to think of work. Your mind never leaves your body, no matter how many things you have to deal with. When you leave meditation, you can do whatever you need to do. Now, we focus on now.

Breath: Focus on breaths that are deep, slow, mindful, and controlled. With each inhalation, you bring maximum oxygen to your body; with each exhalation you relax your entire body. Really pay attention to your breath. This is the way you know how much oxygen you can bring to your body: with a shallow breath, you get less oxygen; with a deeper breath, you get more oxygen; it's pretty much common sense.

Body: Your body needs to be in a comfortable position. If you are not comfortable, you will need to find a way to make yourself comfortable. Your body needs to be completely relaxed from head to toe, including fingers. This is a perfect time to rejuvenate your body with relaxation. Many people don't know how to relax. Many times, when I ask my patients or my students to relax, they tell me, "I thought I *was* relaxed." Your facial muscles also need to be relaxed, including your jaw. Place your tongue behind your upper teeth, on the upper palate, which keeps the roof of your mouth open.

When you finish your meditation, you will feel much better, calmer and more relaxed. You will experience diminished anger and become more productive.

If you use qigong for meditation, you get "two for the price of one"—meditation and body motion. I really enjoy using qigong for my meditation. It is the first thing I do in the morning: if I have time, I do thirty to sixty minutes (adding tai chi); if I don't have as much time, I do five to fifteen minutes. The days I practice, I feel much more energetic and more productive, and my emotions are much more balanced.

6. Listen to relaxing music. If you can remember, turn on relaxing music after work while driving home or when you get home. Music is very healing. It calms your brain and allows your mind to relax by following the beautiful melody. In the morning you can listen to rock and roll or other fast-paced music; but in the after-noon or evening, fast-paced music may make you agitated. If you are sleepy while driving home, you can use fast, rhythmic music to elevate your energy. In the evening, relaxing music helps sleep. You can listen to relaxing music one hour before bed. It helps many people to sleep, and it is worth a try.

7. Practice writing things down. It is very beneficial to get in the habit of writing down, each evening, the work you have to do the next day. When you write things down, you don't need to think about them anymore. I call this technique "unload your mind: use only your eyes." It helps me a lot; I will know what to do because everything is on the paper, and I don't need to worry that I might forget the thing I have to do or have to say the next day. I don't have to think anymore. Writing things down helps avoid making circles in the mind, which is totally useless. Also, the next day, when you accomplish the things you wrote down and cross them off the list, you feel so good. Some people prefer to use technology, such as a smartphone. The problem is, if you misplace the phone, or the phone battery runs out, it won't work. Also, it takes more time and strains your eyes to put the notes in the smartphone. A piece of paper, to me, is much easier, and easy to discard after I complete the work. But it is totally your choice.

8. Practice letting go. This is a very important and beneficial practice, but many people have trouble with it. If you are unable to let go of negativity and tension, the body and mind store these negative emotions and that causes chronic stress. Chronic stress is the number one cause of illnesses. Chronic stress causes insomnia, heart disease, depression, hypertension, high cholesterol, low energy, low immune function, memory loss, headaches, digestive issues, and more. To remove chronic stress, you will need to have a daily practice of detachment.

To practice efficiently, you first need to realize what thoughts you are holding in your head that are troubling you or making you tense and uneasy. Once you know which exact thoughts are troublesome, ask yourself, What I am doing to myself? Why do I need to keep thinking these things? Why am I still living in the past? Why can't I live in the now, today and tomorrow? You then tell yourself, I am going to live smart and not let these affect my life from now on. I am going to move forward, not backward. I can do this! Once you have these affirmations, most of the time you can let the useless thoughts go from your mind right away. When they return, which is very common, you will practice these affirmations again. After many times, you will feel your thoughts are easier to control and easier to let go. Eventually, you don't think about these old memories anymore.

To be able to ease your mind or rest your mind is part of healing. Practicing qigong helps ease the mind and relax the body. That is why qigong is considered a healing exercise.

9. Practice qigong/tai chi. I love qigong and tai chi. They are the best exercises for healing and prevention. They are moving meditation, an internal energy workout; they make your body more agile and flexible; they make your body and limbs more coordinated; they make you feel good right way; and they make you more grounded and balanced. Tai chi and qigong practice provide so many health benefits; that is why the world is attracted to these amazing exercises. In every country and city you can find people doing these exercises.

The East/West Approach to Insomnia

- **Ensure a safe and comfortable sleeping environment.**
- **Turn off all electronics at least one hour before bed.**
- **Avoid stimulants such as caffeine later in the day.**
- **Only lie down when you are actually sleepy.**
- **Get out of bed at the same time every morning.**
- **Engage in adequate cardiovascular exercise during the day.**
- **Meditate, perform qigong in the evening, or do both.**
- **See your doctor if your insomnia persists.**
- **Consider acupuncture and herbal formulas.**

CHAPTER 5

Qigong for Anxiety, Depression, and Insomnia

T HE TERM *QIGONG* IS COMPOSED OF TWO WORDS. The first, "qi" has been translated as the "life energy" or "vital force" within the body. "Gong" has been translated as "work" or "mastery." Together, the word qigong can be interpreted as "energy work" or the act of mastering one's vital force. Qigong is a healing practice that combines breath control with concentration of the mind. There are many forms of qigong, but all fall within two basic types: passive and active. Passive qigong is performed seated or lying down and resembles the stances we associate with meditation; it is also known as internal qigong or nei gong. In the active form of qigong, breath control and focused attention are combined with specific movements to create a type of moving meditation. Active qigong, also known as external qigong or wei gong, is similar to tai chi and yoga.

The practice of qigong is an ancient one. These exercises have been known by several names over the centuries, including Dao-Yin, "leading and guiding the energy."[1] Earlier, we discussed the silk texts that were discovered in the Mawangdui tombs in 1973, which date back to 168 BCE. A chart was found among these texts that depicts the Dao-Yin postures. The Dao-Yin Tu ("Dao-Yin Illustrations") consists of four rows

---

1. Kenneth S. Cohen, *The Way of Qigong: The Art and Science of Chinese Energy Healing* (New York: Ballantine Books, 1997), 13.

of eleven postures, forty-four in all. In these illustrations, the roots of most modern qigong practices can be found; they also include descriptions of the stances, instructions for the movements, and indications for the use of each exercise. Certain Dao-Yin exercises were deemed valuable in treating low back pain and painful knees; others were indicated for gastrointestinal disorders; and still others were designated to treat anxiety. This demonstrates that not only were Dao-Yin exercises prescribed as a medical therapy, but ancient physicians also appreciated the utility of this type of qigong practice in the treatment of emotional disharmony.[2]

As old as qigong is, its development was likely influenced by the older Indian practice of yoga. The earliest known documentation of yoga was found in the Indus Valley and dates back 5,000 years. Two millennia later, in approximately 1000 BCE, the Upanishads were written. These commentaries emphasize the personal, experiential nature of the journey toward spirituality and elucidate many basic yoga teachings, promoting an understanding of the principles of karma, chakras, meditation, and prana.[3] In India, the vital life force is known as prana, and pranayama is the cultivation of the life force through breath control. By breathing with intention, the prana is moved through the nadi (channels). The intersections of important nadi are called chakras. There are many similarities between this system of energy management and that of qigong and Eastern medicine. Qigong requires the same attention and control of the breath and the movement of qi through channels of the body. Interestingly, the locations of many important acupuncture points correspond to the positions of the chakras.

Yoga and tai chi have many benefits, but we feel that qigong is the best practice if you are new to these Eastern healing arts, especially if you have any physical limitations that prevent prolonged standing or

---

2. Ibid.

3. Jennie Lee, *True Yoga: Practicing with the Yoga Sutras for Happiness and Spiritual Fulfillment* (Woodbury, MN: Llewellyn Worldwide, 2016), 7.

impede your ability to move between standing and lying positions. Whether you practice nei gong or wei gong, the regulation of the essential components is related and inseparable: the body, the breath, the mind (thoughts), the qi, and the spirit (emotions).[4] The purpose of regulating and strengthening these components is to achieve good health and longevity.

These related and inseparable elements can also be understood, in a traditional sense, as the Three Treasures: *jing, qi,* and *shen.* In Eastern medicine, the Three Treasures are considered the root of life. The *jing* is often translated as "essence" and, in a Western sense, is akin to your genetic constitution, a fundamental substance that is intimately involved with reproduction, growth, and development of the body from birth to death. As we discussed previously, *qi* has been described as the vital, dynamic force that animates the body. It could be considered the current that runs the motor of our metabolism and drives every aspect of our bodily functions. The term *shen* is harder to translate; for our purposes, it can be thought of as our mind or spirit. Depending on the context, the word *shen* can mean immortal, god, spirit, mind, or soul.[5]

By practicing qigong, we can strengthen the Three Treasures. Because the *jing, qi,* and *shen* are inseparable, each supports and fortifies the others, leading to better physical and emotional health and well-being.

It is beyond the scope of this book to have a complete discussion of the metaphysical aspects of qigong,[6] but an in-depth understanding of qigong is not necessary for you to begin your practice. What is necessary?

---

4. Michael M. Zanoni, *Healing Resonance Qi Gong and Hamanaleo Meditation: Introductory Comments,* https://docs.wixstatic.com/ugd/9371b9_1f315b1505394b7bb b6ceeb9dc4272a6.pdf.

5. Jwing-Ming Yang, *The Root of Chinese Qigong: Secrets for Health, Longevity and Enlightenment,* 2nd ed. (Wolfeboro, NH: YMAA Publication Center, 1989), 28.

6. For the interested reader, many excellent books on this topic are listed in the Recommended Reading and Resources section.

You must focus attention on your breath and be aware of the flow of qi as you move your body with intention.

Qigong is a journey. The goal is not perfection, but incremental improvement in physical, emotional, and spiritual well-being. Patience and persistence are the key to receiving the many benefits of qigong.

Benefits of Qigong

Qigong practice benefits all parts of the body, including all the organ systems and the brain.[7] Here we discuss some examples of these benefits.

Nervous System Benefits

Qigong offers huge benefits to both our central nervous system and our peripheral nervous system. Qigong helps concentration, improves mental alertness, and helps control emotion. Practice also helps preserve vision and hearing as the body ages.

Cardiovascular Benefits

Qi is dynamic. It performs like a motor that pushes the blood where it should go. If a person's qi is strong and circulates well in the body, their blood will also circulate well. If a person's qi is stagnant or weak, it will cause blood stagnation, which, according to Eastern medical theory, can cause heart disease. Qigong contributes to better heart health by regulating the autonomic nervous system. In particular, these exercises activate the vagus nerve, which is a great way to preserve heart energy, normalize cardiac arrhythmias, and maintain normal blood pressure.

Respiratory Benefits

Through deep and slow breathing, more oxygen goes into the lungs. Slow and deep breathing also activates the parasympathetic (calming) part

---

7. Dr. Aihan Kuhn, *True Brain Fitness: Preventing Brain Aging through Body Movement* (Wolfeboro, NH: YMAA Publication Center, 2017), 11.

of the autonomic nervous system. Recall that the nervous system interfaces with the immune system. This process helps the functioning of all cells through proper oxygenation while also improving defensive energy—which in Western medicine we call the "respiratory immune system"—through modulation of the immune system. The lining of the nose, throat, lungs, gut, and urinary tract all contain immunoglobulin A (IgA). IgA is an antibody in the respiratory tract, which protects it from various germs and pathogens and acts as the first line of defense against bacteria and viruses. If the respiratory immune system is strong, immunoglobulin A (IgA) can fight germs, allowing less opportunity for colds and other respiratory infections to take hold; this is why those who practice qigong generally have fewer illnesses.

Gastrointestinal (GI) Benefits

Qigong can improve stomach and spleen energy, which is related to digestion and absorption. From a Western perspective, qigong regulates the vagus nerve, which also controls digestion. With regular practice, digestive enzymes and digestive movement stay balanced through vagus nerve regulation.

Musculoskeletal Benefits

Once the circulation of the qi and blood are improved, muscles receive more oxygen and blood—the muscles become more resilient, more toned, and stronger. Muscle aging is delayed, and joints become more flexible. Overall, we can maintain a younger body even though we are going through the aging process.

Metabolism and Endocrine System Benefits

Balanced qi also helps balance the body's organ systems, which helps balance metabolism and the endocrine system. Here again, these benefits are due to the effect that qigong has on our nervous systems. The central and peripheral nervous systems are intimately connected to the endocrine and immune systems. Neuroendocrine-immune dysfunction can explain a variety of Western diagnoses, such as chronic fatigue syndrome, also known as myalgic encephalomyelitis.

Immune System Benefits

Qigong maintains normal immune function.[8] We have already discussed how these exercises can improve respiratory immunity to help keep infections at bay. For cancer patients, a healthy immune system can help prevent secondary infections during treatment. For those without cancer, a healthy immune system can identify precancerous cells and destroy them.

By balancing the sympathetic and parasympathetic nervous systems, qigong also balances the immune system, so that the immune system is neither too weak nor too strong. A weak immune system will result in recurrent infections. An overly aggressive immune system may result in autoimmune diseases like rheumatoid arthritis. In autoimmune diseases, the immune system turns against the body and attacks normal tissue. Qigong and tai chi help keep the immune system balanced.

Other benefits of qigong include delayed aging, improved balance, reduced risk of falling and injury, and improved memory.[9]

Now it is time to begin your journey and start your qigong practice.

---

8. Dr. Aihan Kuhn, *Simple Chinese Medicine: A Beginner's Guide to Natural Healing and Well-Being* (Wolfeboro, NH: YMAA Publication Center, 2009), 137.

9. For further reading, please see Recommended Reading and Resources at the end of this book.

Qigong Exercises for the Mind

1. Pray for Peace

This movement helps to center your energy and connect arm channels, which include the heart meridian, small intestine meridian, lung meridian, large-intestine meridian, pericardium meridian, and triple-burner meridian.

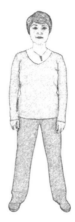

Begin with the feet about shoulder width apart.

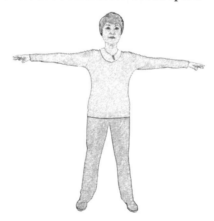

Take a slow, deep breath as you raise your arms out from the sides of your body.

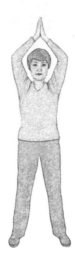

Continue to raise your arms above your head. Put your palms and fingers together.

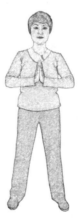

Exhale slowly while moving your hands, palms still together, down to the front of your chest.

Continue to breathe slowly and deeply while keeping this position, and imagine the energy from the earth going up through your feet and then up through your body as you inhale. Exhale as you envision the energy going through your arms, connecting the left and right hands through the fingers. Focus your mind on an inner circle of this energy path.

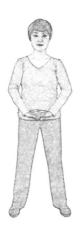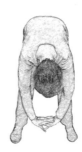

After several breaths, inhale as you interlock your fingers. Exhale as you bend forward, and move your hands down toward the floor. Relax the body. Take another breath.

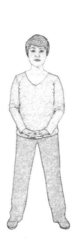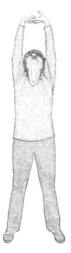

Slowly raise yourself upright, curling your spine up one vertebra at a time, palms facing up. Raise your body to stand straight. At the same time, lift your palms. Inhale as you push your palms up as high as you can. Keep your fingers interlocked.

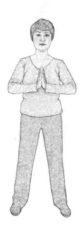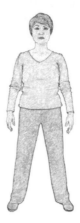

Take another breath. Exhale as you unlock your fingers and put your fingers and thumbs together with your palms together. Keeping your palms together, move your hands to chest level and hold this position for another breath or two. Relax your arms and hands to your sides. Repeat this whole sequence four times.

2. Head Roll

This movement helps open congestion or blockages in the neck area. In many cases, these blockages can disrupt sleep and cause other problems.

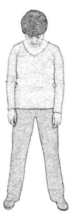

With your head upright, take a deep breath. Exhale as you move your head downward with your chin toward your chest.

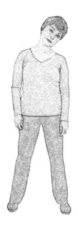 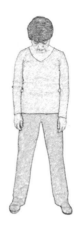

Inhale as you roll your head to the left, and end with your ear over the left shoulder. Exhale as you roll your head down to the front.

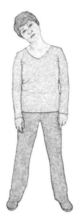 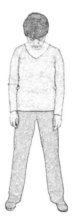

Inhale and roll your head to the right, ending with the ear over the right shoulder. Exhale as you roll your head down to the front.

Repeat these 4 to 8 times, depending on how comfortable you are.

3. Move Qi to the Upper *Dan Tian*

Dan tian means "elixir field" or "sea of qi." These areas are focal points that can create and store qi, acting like reservoirs. The body has three *dan tian*: upper, middle, and lower. The upper *dan tian* is on the head, between the eyes; the middle *dan tian* is on the middle of the breastbone at the level of the fourth rib; and the lower *dan tian* is several inches below the navel, on the midline. This exercise helps move qi to the upper *dan tian*, which influences the mind.

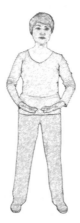

Begin with your feet shoulder width apart. Gather your hands in the front of the lower abdomen, with your palms facing up.

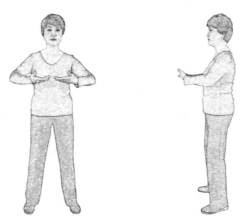

Inhale slowly as you move your palms up to the level of your upper chest.

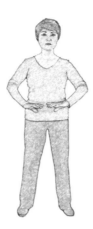

Exhale slowly as you turn your palms facing down. Move them down in front of your body to the level of your lower abdomen.

Repeat the same process for a total of 8 times.

4. Bring Qi to the Eyes

This movement makes use of the *laogong* point in the center of the palm. The *laogong* point is considered a qi gate, meaning that, from this point, the qi in the body can more easily connect with the qi around you. When you place your *laogong* point to your eye, you are moving energy to your eye. The purpose of this exercise is to clear your vision. With regular practice, your vision may improve.

You can either sit or stand, whichever is most comfortable.

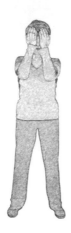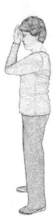

Place your palms in front of your eyes, about 1 to 3 inches away from your face. Hold this position for two minutes, or as long as you are comfortable.

Imagine you are constantly moving the energy from the center of your palms to your eyes. You may feel the heat in your palms go to your eyes. Your breaths are even and slow. With every exhalation you move energy to your eyes. Make sure to relax your shoulders and your entire body.

Repeat once.

5. Neck Massage, Head Massage, and Face Massage

This exercise is used to remove stagnation, promote circulation, remove pain, and nurture the body. Note that in the left-hand side figures, the hand is flat. Then, in the right-hand side figures, the fingers are curved. Apply firm pressure between the fingers and palm to work the muscles.

You can either sit or stand to perform this exercise.

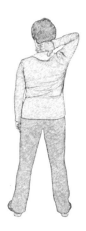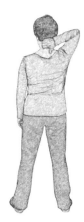

Place your right hand behind your neck. Use the four fingers of your right hand to massage the left side of the neck by grabbing toward the midline of the neck.

Try to massage the deep layer of your neck muscles using your fingertips. You may feel the tightness as you massage the deep muscle of the neck. This should feel very good.

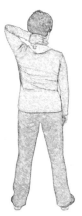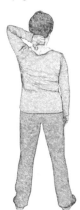

After about thirty seconds, or a bit longer if you are comfortable, change hands. Using your left hand, use the four fingers to massage the right side of your neck.

Use your fingertips to massage the deep layer of your neck muscle on the right side of your neck. You can change sides again as you wish.

6. Bend Forward and Relax

This movement really helps open the bladder channel, which is the longest in the body. The bladder channel contains all the points that strongly influence the internal organs of the body. This channel has a close relationship to the nervous system and the nerves that travel from the spinal cord to the internal organs. The points on the bladder channel that are assigned to each organ correspond to the anatomic location of the nerves that modulate the function of that organ. For example, the point on the bladder channel that influences the function of the heart is located at the level of the spinal column where this nerve travels from the spinal cord toward the heart. By opening the bladder channel, all the organs will benefit.

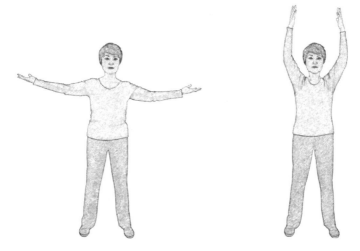

Begin with your feet shoulder width apart. Inhale as you raise your arms up from the side of the body, palms facing up. Exhale as your palms face each other while you reach above your head.

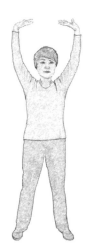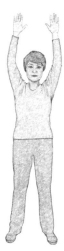

Inhale as you turn your palms upward and push them up as high as you can.

Exhale as you relax your palms.

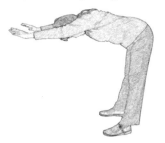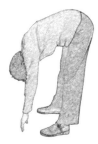

Lower your arms in the front of the body with your palms facing forward, then downward. Continue this motion while bending forward until your fingers touch the floor.

You are bending as low as you can while still feeling comfortable. Relax your arms and upper body and breathe deeply and naturally.

Your mind is focused on total relaxation: arms, shoulder, upper body, lower back. Your knees can be either straight or slightly bent, whatever feels comfortable. With each inhalation, you imagine that the energy goes through your lower back, starting from your feet. With each exhalation you move the energy from the lower back through your body to your fingertips and then connect with the earth's energy.

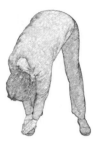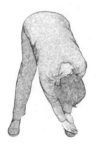

After four deep breaths, while keeping this posture, move your hands over your right foot for one breath cycle. Move your hands over your left foot for one breath cycle.

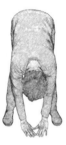

Move your hands to the middle, between your feet.

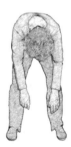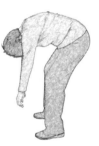

Slowly roll up your body by raising your lower back, upper back, shoulders, neck and head, until standing. Repeat this whole sequence twice.

7. Draw Energy from Earth

There are three energies in the universe: heaven, earth, and human. In order to be more grounded, we want to be more connected to the energy of the earth. As you inhale, you draw energy from the earth. When you exhale, energy moves back to the earth through your body and helps you feel more grounded.

Begin with your feet at shoulder width or wider, depending on your comfort level. Relax your shoulders and upper body.

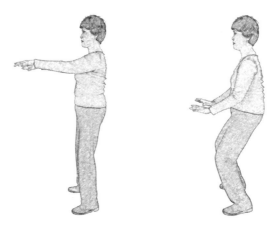

Inhale without lifting your shoulders. Raise the body, and move your arms and hands in the front of the body to shoulder level. Exhale as you sink the body, shoulders, elbows, forearms, wrists, and hands. The knees are unlocked or bent, and the body is relaxed. Perform this movement 8 times.

Visualize the energy from the earth going through your feet, legs, lower abdomen, chest, arms, and hands. Exhale as you bend both legs. Visualize the energy sinking back into the earth.

This movement is similar to tai chi preparation, which is the beginning of tai chi practice, but here there is more focus on drawing qi from the earth.

8. Lotus Palm

This is a meditation pose. By focusing your mind on your breath and posture, you center on your energy, clear your mind, and concentrate on the present moment. As we have discussed previously, meditation confers huge benefits to the body.

This movement requires that you either kneel or sit on the floor. You could even sit on a chair if you wish.

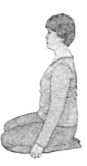

Sit on your heels with your lower back relaxed.

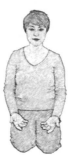

Place your hands on your lap, above your knees, palms up. Focus your mind on your palms. Feel the heat in the center of your palms.

With each inhalation, feel more energy go into your palms and your arms; with each exhalation the energy moves up your arms and goes to into your body. Continue to focus on your palms and the energy flow. You feel peaceful, calm, and comfortable. You feel the energy flow smoothly in your body.

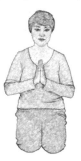

After several minutes of breathing and focusing, inhale, raising your palms. Exhale and place your palms together in front of the body, like a prayer position. Stay in this position for several breaths, several minutes.

You have now completed your practice.

CHAPTER 6

General Principles of Self-Healing

U LTIMATELY, THE SUCCESSFUL TREATMENT OF ANXIETY, depression, and insomnia depends on consistent self-care. Even if you are taking medications for these conditions, you must be attentive to your body, mind, and spirit on a daily basis. Medications must be taken regularly without skipping doses, and doctors' appointments should be kept. Your health-care provider can do a lot for you, from arriving at a correct diagnosis to arranging specialty and support services.

But you can do even more for yourself. We all know that eating nutritious foods, not smoking, exercising regularly, sleeping adequately, and managing stress levels can lead to a healthier life. In fact, the World Health Organization (WHO) and Centers for Disease Control (CDC) have determined that if people would exercise more, eat better, and not smoke, 40 percent of cancers and 80 percent of adult-onset diabetes and heart disease could be prevented.[1] Sleep deprivation and life stress have each been shown to contribute to the incidence of chronic illness, so sleeping well and managing stress can decrease your risk of such diseases.

Taking care of yourself requires determination. Every day you will be faced with choices about what foods to buy and how to cook them,

---

1. Kenneth Thorpe and Jonathan Lever, "Prevention: The Answer to Curbing Chronically High Health Care Costs (Guest Opinion)," *Kaiser Health News*, May 24, 2011, http://www.kaiserhealthnews.org/Columns/2011/May/052411thorpelever.aspx.

how much to eat, and how to exercise and for how long. You also make choices about whether to go to sleep at a reasonable hour or stay up and surf the internet. You choose whether to manage your stress by using meditative practices or dangerous habits such as smoking or excessive alcohol consumption. Every decision you make matters. Your doctor can give you advice, but ultimately, you must decide for yourself and act on those decisions. No one else can do it for you.

If you have already established these healthy habits, congratulations! You are stacking the odds in your favor. The likelihood that you will develop a lifestyle-related chronic illness is at least half what it would be otherwise. As we have seen, even conditions like anxiety, depression, and insomnia can be improved through lifestyle modification.

If you feel there is room for improvement in the way you eat, exercise, and manage your stress, now is the time to gear up and get going. In our first book, *True Wellness: How to Combine the Best of Western and Eastern Medicine for Optimal Health*, we devoted a whole chapter to the process of change, setting goals, and taking action to achieve those objectives. We have found that one of the most useful tools you can use to establish new habits is a checklist. There is nothing particularly glamorous or high-tech about a checklist, but for many people, it is invaluable. With a checklist, you can see concretely what you have or have not done during the course of your week. If you plan to practice qigong three times a week, you can see as the days pass whether you will meet that goal. If you are honest, you will see the number of times you meditated or went to the gym, how many vegetables you ate, or how much water you drank. Many people, when they start using a checklist, are astonished at their own lapses. We often convince ourselves that we are doing all we can to achieve optimal health, when really we are falling short of the mark. This sort of wishful thinking is common.

The beauty of a checklist is that it gives you a systematic way of changing your behavior and developing consistency. The checklist has become integral in air-traffic safety and in hospital operating rooms. Its use has improved outcomes in these industries where lives hang in the balance. It is not being too melodramatic to say that both the quality and quantity of your years on earth depend on establishing habits that maximize your physical, emotional, and spiritual health.

Decades of medical research show that most chronic illnesses are lifestyle driven and that the underlying physiological problem in these conditions is chronic inflammation. Many studies demonstrate that eating a minimally processed plant-based diet; meditating; practicing qigong, tai chi, or yoga; exercising regularly; and getting adequate sleep all decrease chronic inflammation. Using the True Wellness Checklist can effectively support your shift toward a healthy lifestyle, decrease chronic inflammation, and reduce your risk of developing many chronic conditions.

The True Wellness Checklist

Instructions for Use

The True Wellness Checklist is a compilation of recommended actions that are associated with optimal health. These actions form the basis of disease prevention in both Eastern and Western medical systems. Meditation, qigong, cardiovascular exercise, and resistance training should be incorporated into everyone's healing plan. Optimizing your sleep can improve your physical and emotional health. As we have seen throughout this book, anxiety and depression can disrupt your sleep, but the reverse is also true: poor sleep can disrupt mental health. This is why we have included in this version of the True Wellness Checklist measures you can take to improve the quality and quantity of your sleep.

Many people have food sensitivities, allergies, or individual preferences; therefore, the dietary recommendations on the checklist form the essentials of a vegan regimen. You can add servings of meat, fish, or dairy, depending on your tastes or requirements. The majority of your food should be plant based. If you do eat animal products, your plate should be filled three-quarters with plants and only one-quarter with animal protein. Choose whole foods over processed foods. Minimize sweets, but on occasion enjoy chocolate made of at least 70 percent cacao.

Approximate serving sizes

Vegetables	1 cup raw vegetables, ½ cup cooked vegetables
Fruit	1 medium piece raw fruit, ½ cup canned fruit, ¼ cup dried fruit
Nuts	⅓ cup
Beans/Legumes	½ cup cooked
Whole Grains	1 slice bread, ½ cup cooked grains, 1 ounce dry cereal
Red Meat, Poultry	cooked, roughly the same size as a deck of cards
Fish	uncooked, 8 ounces (no more than 3x/week because of heavy metals)
Dairy	1 cup yogurt, 1 cup milk, 2 ounces of cheese
Eggs	1 egg
Oils	extra virgin olive oil for cooking, flaxseed oil for dressings

True Wellness Checklist

	Daily Practice	Day 1	Day 2	Day 3	Day 4	Day 5	Day 6	Day 7
sleep	• Wake up at the same time every day	☐	☐	☐	☐	☐	☐	☐
	• Meditate daily	☐	☐	☐	☐	☐	☐	☐
	• No caffeine after 3:00 p.m.	☐	☐	☐	☐	☐	☐	☐
	• No naps after 3:00 p.m.	☐	☐	☐	☐	☐	☐	☐
	• Exercise no later than 3 hours before bed	☐	☐	☐	☐	☐		
	• No electronics 1–2 hours before bed	☐	☐	☐	☐	☐	☐	☐
	• Keep bedroom cool and dark	☐	☐	☐	☐	☐	☐	☐
	• Go to bed at the same time every night, if sleepy	☐	☐	☐	☐	☐	☐	☐
	• If not asleep in 15 minutes, engage in relaxing activity without electronics, then lie down again when sleepy*	☐	☐	☐	☐	☐	☐	☐
food	• Vegetables (4–6 servings daily)	☐	☐	☐	☐	☐	☐	☐
	• Fruit (3–4 servings daily)	☐	☐	☐	☐	☐	☐	☐
	• Nuts (1/3 cup daily)	☐	☐	☐	☐	☐	☐	☐
	• Beans/Legumes (1–2 servings daily)	☐	☐	☐	☐	☐	☐	☐
	• Grains (3–4 servings daily)	☐	☐	☐	☐	☐	☐	☐
	• Water (8 glasses daily)	☐	☐	☐	☐	☐	☐	☐
	• Protein of choice	☐	☐	☐	☐	☐	☐	☐
move-ment	• Cardiovascular exercise (2–5x/week)	☐	☐	☐	☐	☐	☐	☐
	• Resistance training (2–5x/week)	☐	☐	☐	☐	☐	☐	☐
	• Qigong or Tai Chi (5–7x/week)	☐	☐	☐	☐	☐	☐	☐
fun	• At least one 15-minute activity every day, simply for your own enjoyment	☐	☐	☐	☐	☐	☐	☐

* Suggested activities: read a book (an old-fashioned hard copy), meditate, do restorative stretching or qigong, have a warm bath or shower, listen to calming music, breathe in a pattern where your exhalation is about twice as long as your inhalation.

Conclusion

THE MARK OF TRUE HEALTH is not maintaining a perfect status quo—that is an impossible task. There will always be problems in life, health problems included. Health problems may arise because of genetic predisposition, early adverse life events, disregard for emotional and physical self-care, socioeconomic disadvantage, catastrophe, or plain old bad luck. Just when you feel you have things under control again, you may experience another setback. Everyone has gone through dark days, to one degree or another.

True health is resilience, the ability to adapt to external and internal stressors and use every means available to speed your recovery. We strongly recommend incorporating Eastern techniques of meditation and movement, acupuncture and herbs, into your Western therapeutic plan for anxiety, depression, or insomnia. These modalities will bolster your sense of well-being and calm, easing the pain and stress of chronic illness. Our patients report that these interventions improve their sleep and strength. With this newfound energy, they are better able to care for themselves. They exercise more often, which enhances their mood and sleep. They eat more nutritiously, which improves many of their bodily functions. They become more determined to examine their relationships, resolve current and past disharmonies, and tackle detrimental addictions such as smoking, excessive drinking, or substance abuse, all of which strongly influence emotional health and sleep.

Consistently weaving Eastern therapies into Western care will give you an advantage when an unexpected stressor crosses your path, as it inevitably will. You will have the tools in place to more easily weather the storm and gain confidence in your capabilities and increasing resilience. This is the beauty of integrative medicine. Each component supports the other, magnifying the positive effects synergistically.

We wish you every success on your journey.

Acknowledgments

I N THE PROCESS OF CO-WRITING THIS BOOK SERIES, we have had many supporters. We would like to take this opportunity to thank all our advisers, reviewers, illustrators, and editors, who keep this project moving in the right direction. At YMAA Publication Center we are grateful for the efforts of publisher David Ripianzi, managing editor T. G. LaFredo, production manager Tim Comrie, illustrator and designer Axie Breen, and publicist Barbara Langley. At Westchester Publishing Services, we would like to thank editor Deborah Grahame-Smith and copyeditor Susan Campbell for fine-tuning the manuscript.

Special thanks go to Jeanne Heroux for her enthusiasm and willingness to write the foreword to this book. Her dedication to the integration of Eastern and Western medicine is a wonderful benefit to her patients.

To all these supporters and our families, to Dr. Kuhn's students and fans from the United States and around the world, to members of the Tai Chi & Qi Gong Healing Institute, and to you, the reader, we recognize and appreciate your trust, your encouragement, and your passion for mind-body healing. Together, we will build a peaceful world.

Recommended Reading and Resources

Organizations

American Academy of Medical Acupuncture: https://www.medicalacupuncture.org/Find-an-Acupuncturist

American Academy of Sleep Medicine: www.sleepeducation.org

American Psychiatric Association: https://www.psychiatry.org

Anxiety and Depression Association of America (ADAA): https://adaa.org

National Certification Commission for Acupuncture and Oriental Medicine: www.nccaom.org/find-a-practitioner-directory

National Suicide Prevention Lifeline: call 1-800-273-TALK, 1-800-273-8255, available 24/7, https://www.suicidepreventionlifeline.org

Books

Blackburn, Elizabeth, and Elissa Epel. *The Telomere Effect: A Revolutionary Approach to Living Younger, Healthier, Longer.* New York: Grand Central Publishing, 2017.

Brogan, Kelly, and Kristen Loberg. *A Mind of Your Own: The Truth about Depression and How Women Can Heal Their Bodies to Reclaim Their Lives.* New York: Harper Wave, 2016.

Cohen, Kenneth. *The Way of Qigong: The Art and Science of Chinese Energy Healing.* New York: Ballantine Books, 1997.

Doidge, Norman. *The Brain that Changes Itself.* New York: Viking/Penguin, 2007.

Doidge, Norman. *The Brain's Way of Healing.* New York: Penguin, 2015.

Harris, Dan. *10% Happier: How I Tamed the Voice in My Head, Reduced Stress without Losing My Edge, and Found Self-Help that Actually Works—A True Story.* New York: HarperCollins, 2014.

Helms, Joseph. *Getting to Know You: A Physician Explains How Acupuncture Helps You Be the Best You.* Berkeley, CA: Medical Acupuncture Publishers, 2007.

Kaptchuk, Ted. *The Web that Has No Weaver: Understanding Chinese Medicine.* New York: McGraw-Hill, 2000.

Keown, Daniel. *The Spark in the Machine: How the Science of Acupuncture Explains the Mysteries of Western Medicine.* London: Singing Dragon, 2014.

Kuhn, Aihan. *Brain Fitness: The Easy Way of Keeping Your Mind Sharp through Qigong*. Wolfeboro, NH: YMAA Publication Center, 2017.

Kuhn, Aihan. *Natural Healing with Qigong: Therapeutic Qigong*. Wolfeboro, NH: YMAA Publication Center, 2004.

Kuhn, Aihan. *Simple Chinese Medicine: A Beginner's Guide to Natural Healing and Well-Being*. Wolfeboro, NH: YMAA Publication Center, 2009.

Kuhn, Aihan. *Tai Chi for Depression: A 10-Week Program to Empower Yourself and Beat Depression*. Wolfeboro, NH: YMAA Publication Center, 2017.

Kuhn, Aihan. *Tai Chi in 10 Weeks: Beginner's Guide: A Proven Step-by-Step Plan for Integrating the Physical and Psychological Benefits of Tai Chi in to Your Life*. Wolfeboro, NH: YMAA Publication Center, 2017.

Kurosu, Catherine, and Aihan Kuhn. *True Wellness: How to Combine the Best of Western and Eastern Medicine for Optimal Health*. Wolfeboro, NH: YMAA Publication Center, 2018.

Lee, Jennie. *Breathing Love: Meditation in Action*. Woodbury, MN: Llewellyn Worldwide, 2018.

Lee, Jennie. *True Yoga: Practicing with the Yoga Sutras for Happiness and Spiritual Fulfillment*. Woodbury, MN: Llewellyn Worldwide, 2016.

Scheid, Volker, and Hugh MacPherson, editors. *Integrating East Asian Medicine into Contemporary Health Care*. Edinburgh: Churchill Livingstone, Elsevier, 2012.

Walker, Matthew. *Why We Sleep: Unlocking the Power of Sleep and Dreams*. New York: Scribner, 2017.

Weil, Andrew. *You Can't Afford to Get Sick: Your Guide to Optimum Health and Health Care*. New York: Plume, 2009.

Yang, Jwing-Ming. *The Root of Chinese Qigong: Secrets for Health, Longevity and Enlightenment*. 2nd ed. Wolfeboro, NH: YMAA Publication Center, 1989.

Glossary

Accreditation Commission for Acupuncture and Oriental Medicine (ACAOM). The national agency, recognized by the United States Department of Education (USDoED), that accredits master's-level programs in acupuncture and Oriental medicine, ensuring that such programs meet the standards for education set by Congress.

acupuncture. A system of medicine that involves inserting fine metal needles into specific anatomic locations to treat a variety of illnesses and conditions. Derived from the Latin *acus* (needle) and puncture.

American Academy of Medical Acupuncture (AAMA). A society, founded in 1987, of medical doctors (MDs) and osteopaths (DOs) who have undergone training in acupuncture in order to incorporate this modality into conventional health care.

American Board of Medical Acupuncture (ABMA). An independent entity within the AAMA, established in 2000, to conduct examinations of candidates seeking certification in medical acupuncture in order to maintain high standards for the profession.

American Medical Association (AMA). A professional association of medical doctors (MDs) and osteopaths (DOs) founded in 1847. The stated mission of the AMA is to "promote the art and science of medicine and the betterment of public health."

***Ben Cao Gang Mu* (*Compendium of Materia Medica*).** An encyclopedic medical volume, written in the sixteenth century CE by Li Shi-Zhen, a prominent physician in the Ming dynasty, detailing the herbs and other substances used in Chinese medicine.

Buddhism. A philosophical practice that developed out of the teachings of Siddhartha Gautama in the fifth century BCE and spread from northeastern India through Asia and globally. Gautama became known as Buddha and taught that life is full of suffering, but suffering could be overcome by developing wisdom, integrity, and awareness.

chromosomes. The coiled structures within the nucleus of most cells that contain the genetic information required for life.

Confucianism. The teachings of Confucius, which emphasize correct behavior of the institutions and individuals within society, as well as the cultivation of knowledge and good judgment.

Confucius. A Chinese philosopher, political figure, and educator who lived during the fifth and sixth centuries BCE; his teachings are known as Confucianism.

Dao De Ching. A Chinese text regarding the philosophy of Daoism, attributed to Laozi (see Daoism), which may actually be a compilation of works by later authors.

Daoism. Also known as Taoism. The doctrine of living in harmony with the natural order of the universe, ascribed to the teachings of Laozi, a Chinese philosopher who lived during the sixth century BCE.

DNA (deoxyribonucleic acid). The long double-stranded and twisted chain of organic molecules that constitutes chromosomes. The sequence of the organic molecules acts as a blueprint for the body to create other necessary substances such as proteins and enzymes.

Eastern medicine. A system of medicine that arose in Asia that makes use of herbal remedies, acupuncture, meditation, qigong, and tai chi to improve health. Also known as East Asian medicine or Oriental medicine.

Five Phases. The cosmological scheme that describes interactions among natural phenomena, such as the changing of the seasons, developed in ancient China millennia ago and used in astrology, military strategy, and medicine. Also referred to as the Five Elements (see Wu Xing).

Food and Drug Administration (FDA). An agency of the US Department of Health and Human Services created to ensure that food, drugs, and medical devices are safe and effective. Also, ensures that cosmetic and dietary supplements are safe and labeled properly, and regulates tobacco products.

functional magnetic resonance imaging (fMRI). An imaging technique that employs magnetic and radio waves, used to determine which areas of the brain are most active at the time of the study.

gene. A sequence of DNA that codes for a molecule that has a specific function within a living organism; see DNA.

Huang Di Nei Jing (The Yellow Emperor's Classic of Internal Medicine). An ancient Chinese medical text written approximately during the Han dynasty (206 BCE–220 CE).

Hua Tuo. Famed second-century CE Chinese physician and surgeon who also developed longevity exercises called Five Animal Qigong.

integrative medicine. A branch of conventional Western medicine that is patient-centered and incorporates techniques from other medical systems for which there is good evidence of safety and efficacy.

Journal of the American Medical Association (JAMA). A peer-reviewed medical journal published by the AMA containing research papers, reviews, and editorials that relate to the field of medicine.

Laozi. A Chinese philosopher who lived during the sixth century BCE and developed the doctrine of living in harmony with the natural order of the universe known as Daoism or Taoism.

licensed acupuncturist (LAc). Designation given to a person who has received a license to practice acupuncture from a state medical or professional licensing board. To qualify, that person must have completed a specific amount of training and passed certifying examinations in acupuncture and Eastern medicine.

mind-body medicine. A group of therapeutic practices that engage the mind's capacity to influence bodily functions; examples of these techniques include meditation, relaxation, biofeedback, and hypnosis.

National Certification Commission for Acupuncture and Oriental Medicine (NCCAOM). A nonprofit organization established in 1982 to certify competency of acupuncturists, herbologists, and bodyworkers of Eastern medical disciplines in the United States. The NCCAOM is also involved with recertification, examination development, and continuing education.

neuroplasticity. The ability of the brain to form new connections and pathways in response to learning or training; also known as brain plasticity.

placebo. A substance or intervention that has no active ingredient or expected benefit.

placebo effect. A positive, unexpected benefit seen following administration of a placebo, attributed to the recipient's expectation of benefit, considered a mind-body interaction.

post-heaven qi. Eastern medicine term for energy (qi) extracted by the body from food and air.

pre-heaven qi. Eastern medicine term for energy (qi) that is inherited from our parents, analogous to genetic constitution in Western medicine.

preventive medicine. A medical specialty that focuses on the prevention of disease, not only in the individual patient but also in the community and population at large. A combination of clinical medicine and public health.

PubMed. A free search engine that can be used to find abstracts and articles on life sciences and biomedical subjects, maintained by the National Center for Biotechnology Information at the US National Library of Medicine.

qi. Eastern medicine term for the intelligent life force that flows through the body, often described in Western terms as "energy."

qigong. Mental, physical, and breathing exercises that cultivate qi. Related to tai chi (see tai chi).

Silk Road. Ancient trading route between Asia and Europe that traversed Korea, China, India, Persia, and Europe.

Sun Si-Miao. Prolific seventh-century CE Chinese physician and herbalist who wrote two thirty-volume works on the practice of medicine. He was renowned for integrating Daoism with Buddhism and Confucianism and emphasized ethical behavior for physicians.

tai chi. A Chinese martial art form, but also a series of slow, meditative movements that, when performed regularly, can improve health and well-being. Related to qigong (see qigong).

telomerase. An enzyme that adds specific molecules to the ends of telomeres to preserve their length (see telomere).

telomere. The noncoding DNA sequences on the ends of chromosomes that protect the chromosomes and protect the loss of genetic information during DNA transcription.

tui na. A method of Chinese bodywork or massage.

World Health Organization (WHO). An agency of the United Nations, established in 1948, intended to improve international public health.

Wu Xing. Known in English as the Five Phases or Five Elements. The cosmological scheme that describes interactions among natural phenomena, such as the changing of the seasons, developed in ancient China millennia ago and used in astrology, military strategy, and medicine.

yin-yang theory. The theory that states that all phenomena are composed of two opposite conditions or characteristics. These opposites cannot be separated; together, they represent the unified whole.

Index

acupuncture, 17–18, 20–22, 27–35, 37, 39–42, 53–54, 59–60, 71, 91, 98, 100
acupuncture channels, 18, 27–28, 34
acupuncture points, 18, 27, 29, 32, 34, 100
ACUS Foundation, 40
adenosine, 73–74
adrenocorticotrophic hormone (ACTH), 30
aging, 102–104
alcohol, 3–4, 47, 50–51, 63, 71, 77, 80, 88, 121
allopathy, 38, 42
allostasis, 6
allostatic overload, 6–7
alpha waves, 24
alternative, 38
Alzheimer's disease, 24
American Board of Medical Acupuncturists (ABMA), 131
American Hospital Association, 38
amygdala, 7, 48
ancient Greece, 10
antidepressants, 26, 28, 44–46, 49, 51–54, 64, 68, 78
anti-inflammatory action, 26, 30, 81
anxiety, 1–3, 5, 7, 23, 42–44, 46–54, 59–61, 63–66, 69, 71, 77, 79, 81, 83–84, 90, 92, 99–100, 120–121, 125
Anxiety and Depression Association of America (ADAA), 46
asthma, 78

astrocyte, 4
autoimmune diseases, 6, 13, 104
autonomic nervous system, 7, 23, 48, 92, 102–103

bacteria, 11, 103
balance, 1, 5–6, 10, 16–17, 23, 25, 29, 36, 39, 48, 53–56, 60, 62, 64–65, 85, 92, 103–104, 121
Becker, Robert, 31
Ben Cao Gang Mu (Compendium of Materia Medica), 20–21
beta waves, 24
beta-endorphin, 30
bioelectromagnetic, 34
biomedical, 13, 48, 77, 82
biopsychosocial, 14
blue (wavelength) light, 81, 85, 87, 88
bodywork, 39
brain, 2, 4–8, 12, 23–25, 28, 30–32, 36, 44, 48–50, 61–62, 64–67, 72–75, 79–81, 84, 87–88, 94, 96, 102
brain waves, 24, 72
breath, 22–23, 63–64, 86, 92, 95–96, 99–102, 105, 107–108, 116, 118

cancer, 25, 76, 104
cardiovascular disease, 60
Centers for Disease Control (CDC), 72, 120
central nervous system, 7, 28, 44, 85, 92, 102
cerebrospinal fluid, 4

children, 2, 70, 72
cholesterol, 29, 36, 62, 97
chromosomes, 132, 135
chronic disease, 39
chronic inflammation, 6, 23, 26, 60, 79, 122
Claridge and Helman, 35
coffee, 50, 62, 82
cognitive-behavioral therapy, 7, 83
cognitive-behavioral therapy for insomnia (CBT-I), 83
collagen, 32–34
complementary, 38–40, 42, 44, 46, 52–53, 55
cortisol, 29–30, 79
current of injury, 31

Dao De Ching, 17
Dao-Yin, 99–100
Daoism, 14, 17, 54, 70
delta waves, 24
dementia, 4
depression, 1–3, 5, 7, 42–46, 49–54, 59–61, 63–66, 69, 77, 79, 91, 97, 99, 120–122, 125
diabetes, 6, 13, 60, 62, 76, 120
diet, 17–18, 37, 49–50, 54, 60–61, 90, 122
disharmony, 15, 100
dopamine, 29, 49, 51

Eastern medicine, 14–15, 21–22, 26, 38–42, 56, 58–59, 63, 100–101, 121
electricity, 27, 30–31, 33–34
electroencephalography (EEG), 24
electromagnetic fields, 32
elements, 10, 14–15, 22, 101
emotions, 7, 60–63, 65–66, 75, 93–94, 96–97
endocrine system, 103
endorphins, 30, 49
energy, 11, 18, 32, 34, 54, 56, 58–59, 61–67, 69, 71, 91, 96–100, 102–103, 105–106, 111–112, 115, 117–119, 125

exercise, 3, 10, 13, 17–18, 25–26, 37, 39, 42, 44, 49–50, 53, 55, 59, 65, 67–68, 71, 80, 90, 93–94, 98, 100, 110–112, 120–122, 125
experiments, 27, 31

family, 2, 10, 12
fascia, 32–34
Five Phases, 15–17
Food and Drug Administration (FDA), 132
forgiveness, 69
Foster, Russell, 5
functional magnetic resonance imaging (fMRI), 2, 24
functional MRI, 32

GABA (gamma-aminobutyric acid), 29
gene expression, 3
generalized anxiety disorder, 2, 47–49
genes, 3
genetic, 2–3, 13, 44, 48, 101, 125
genome, 12
glial cell, 4
glymphatic system, 4–5
goal, 5, 54, 82, 102, 121
gray matter, 24
Gryffin, Peter Anthony, 25, 26

Han dynasty, 18
Harper, Donald, 17–18
Harvard, 25, 36, 38
healing, 8–10, 21, 26, 29, 31, 38–39, 42, 54–63, 65–69, 71, 89, 96, 98–100, 104, 122
health, 1, 3, 5–6, 8–11, 13–14, 17–18, 22, 24, 26, 31, 36, 38–42, 44, 46, 48, 51–52, 54–55, 60, 63, 66–67, 69, 71, 73, 75–77, 85–87, 90, 98, 101–102, 120–122, 125
health-care costs, 77
heart disease, 6, 13, 62, 75–76, 97, 102, 120

Helms, Joseph, 17, 27, 29, 32, 40
Helms Medical Institute, 40, 143
herbs, 18, 20–21, 26, 38–39, 42, 44,
   58–59, 125
hippocampus, 7
Hippocrates, 10
homeostasis, 6, 29
hormones, 6–7, 23, 32, 48, 62, 79, 84, 91
*Huang Di Nei Jing (The Yellow Emperor's
   Classic of Internal Medicine)*, 18
Hua Tuo, 21
humors, 10
hypertension, 97

immune system, 25, 30, 36, 79, 103–104
Industrial Revolution, 11–12
inflammation, 6, 23, 25–26, 60, 79, 122
insomnia, 2, 52, 59, 62, 65, 75–92, 94,
   97–99, 120–121, 125
integrative medicine, 38, 47, 49, 77, 82,
   126
interstitium, 32–33

jing, 18, 20, 101
*Journal of the American Medical
   Association (JAMA)*, 44

Kaptchuk, Ted, 16, 37
kava, 51–52, 71
Keown, Daniel, 32–33

Langevin, Helene, 25
Laozi, 14, 17
Li, Shi Zhen, 20
licensed acupuncturist (L.Ac.), 22
lifestyle, 3, 13, 38–40, 46, 54, 77, 82,
   121–122
lifestyle changes, 13, 40, 46, 53

magnetic resonance imaging, 2, 24, 29
martial arts, 67–68
Mawangdui tombs (King Ma's Mound),
   17, 99

medical anthropology, 35, 36
medical education, 12
medical research, 13, 122
medical school, 12
medications, 7, 13, 42, 44–46, 48, 51–54,
   58–59, 64, 71–72, 76–79, 82, 86, 90, 120
medicine, 3–4, 10–18, 20–22, 26, 28–31,
   33, 36–42, 47, 49, 54–56, 58–61, 63, 77,
   79, 81–82, 86, 91, 100–101, 103–104,
   121, 126
meditation, 7–8, 22–26, 37, 39, 52, 59, 63,
   91–92, 94–96, 98–101, 118, 122, 125
Mediterranean-type diet, 50
melatonin, 79–82, 85, 87–88
memory, 3, 7, 24, 48, 81, 86, 94, 104
mental illness, 5, 46
met-enkephalin, 30
mind-body interventions, 37
mindfulness, 23, 71
muscles, 23, 25–26, 31, 33, 65, 83, 96, 103,
   112–113

Naiman, Rubin, 77, 82
narcolepsy, 75–76
National Certification Commission for
   Acupuncture and Oriental Medicine
   (NCCAOM), 129, 134
natural killer cells, 30
nerve fibers, 28, 29
nervous system, 7, 23, 28–29, 44, 48, 52,
   85, 92, 102–103, 114
neural system, 27
neurons, 4, 24
neuroplasticity, 134
neurotransmitters, 5–6, 23, 26, 29, 32,
   48, 50–51, 53, 62, 65
Niboyet, 27
noise-reduction approach to insomnia
   (NRAI), 82, 87
non-rapid eye movement sleep (NREM),
   74
norepinephrine, 29, 49, 51
nutrition, 50, 60–61, 80

obesity, 76

obsessive-compulsive disorder (OCD), 43, 47

obstructive sleep apnea, 75–77

omega-3 fatty acids, 50, 71

opioids, 30

pain, 1–2, 25, 28–30, 35, 40, 47, 61–62, 72, 76–77, 79, 82, 90–91, 100, 112, 125

panic disorder, 47

parasympathetic nervous system, 23, 85

patient, 8–10, 12, 14–15, 17, 20, 30, 33, 35–37, 39–42, 46–48, 51, 54, 56, 58, 61, 70, 75–77, 86, 90–91

peripheral nervous system, 102

persistence, 102

pharmaceuticals, 26, 58

phobias, 47

physician, 10, 21–22, 30, 42, 49, 90

placebo, 34–37

placebo effect, 34–35

plants, 20, 26–27, 58, 122

Positive Mind, 64, 66, 68–70

post-heaven qi, 134

post-traumatic stress disorder, 43, 48

pranayama, 100

pre-heaven qi, 134

prefrontal cortex, 7

preventive medicine, 134

psychotherapy, 44, 49, 53

PubMed, 134

qi, 11, 17–18, 20, 23, 33, 56–57, 59, 63–65, 67, 100–103, 109–111, 117

qigong, 8, 22, 25–26, 37, 39, 52, 54, 56, 59, 63–68, 71, 85, 90–92, 96, 98–104, 121–122, 124

randomized controlled trial, 35, 37

rapid eye movement sleep (REM sleep), 74

research, 3–4, 13, 22, 24, 26–27, 29, 31, 35, 37, 40–41, 49, 52, 122

residency, 12

resilience, 125–126

restless leg syndrome, 75–76

risk of falling, 104

Scientific Revolution, 11

self-care, 120, 125

serotonin, 29, 49–52

sham acupuncture, 34–35

shaman, 9

Shang Han Lun (*Treatise on Cold Damage*), 20

Shen, 101

Shen Nong Ben Cao Jing (*The Divine Farmer's Materia Medica*), 20

shift work disorder, 75–76

Silk Road, 21

sleep, 1–5, 8, 10, 13, 24, 26, 31, 42, 62–63, 71–93, 96, 108, 121–122, 125

sleep apnea, 75–77, 80, 84

sleep deprivation, 3–4

sleep hygiene, 83

sleep opportunity, 76

smoking, 120–121, 125

social anxiety disorder, 47

social connections, 71

society, 2, 57, 63, 76

socioeconomic factors, 1, 14

spirituality, 100

St. John's Wort, 52, 71

stress, 1, 6–7, 23, 33, 40, 43, 47–49, 52, 57, 62, 67, 69–71, 79–80, 83, 86, 90, 97, 120–121, 125

stress management, 80

substance P, 29

sugar, 37, 62

Sun, Si-Miao, 21

sympathetic nervous system, 23, 85

tai chi, 8, 22, 25–26, 37, 39, 52, 54, 56, 59, 63–64, 67–68, 71, 85, 91–92, 96, 98–100, 104, 117, 122

Tang dynasty, 20–21

theta waves, 24

Three Treasures, 101
True Wellness Checklist, 122
tui na, 59–60, 91

ultrasound elastography, 29
Unschuld, Paul, 18

valerian, 51–52, 71, 81, 89
vegan diet, 61
vegetarian diet, 60
viruses, 11, 103
vital force, 17, 99
vitalism, 11
vitamin B, 71
vitamins, 51, 61, 71

Walker, Matthew, 73
water, 10, 16, 34, 62–63, 93, 121

well-being, 5, 9–10, 42, 49, 54–55,
    57, 60, 69, 77, 94, 101–102, 104,
    125
Western medicine, 3, 10–13, 33, 38, 41,
    54, 60, 81, 86, 91, 103
World Health Organization (WHO), 41,
    120
Wu Xing, 15, 20

yang, 11, 15, 55–57, 64,
    101
yin, 11, 14–15, 20, 55–57, 64
yin-yang theory, 14, 18, 20, 56
yoga, 8, 22–23, 25–26, 39, 52, 68, 91,
    99–100, 122

Zhang, Zhong Jin, 20
Zhang and Popp, 34

About the Authors

Dr. Catherine Kurosu

Born, raised, and trained in Canada, Dr. Catherine Kurosu graduated from the University of Toronto School of Medicine in 1990. She completed her internship and residency at the same institution and qualified as a specialist in obstetrics and gynecology in 1995. Dr. Kurosu has studied and worked in Canada, the United States, Mexico, and Chile. 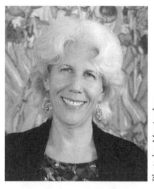 Through her travels, she has learned that there are many ways to approach a problem and that the patient usually understands their illness best. By combining the patient's insight with medical guidance, effective treatment plans can be developed.

In 2006, Dr. Kurosu became a diplomate of the American Board of Holistic Medicine, now known as the American Board of Integrative Holistic Medicine. In 2009, she became certified as a medical acupuncturist through the David Geffen School of Medicine at UCLA and the Helms Medical Institute. Dr. Kurosu became a member of the American Academy of Medical Acupuncture, then a diplomate of the American Board of Medical Acupuncture, which confers this title to practitioners with increasing experience.

Since then, Dr. Kurosu has completed a master of science in Oriental medicine, graduating from the Institute of Clinical Acupuncture and Oriental Medicine in Honolulu. In 2015, she became a licensed acupuncturist and in 2018 became a diplomate in Oriental medicine through the National Certification Commission for Acupuncture and Oriental Medicine.

Photo by: Monica Lau

Dr. Kurosu now lives on Oʻahu with her husband, Rob, and daughter, Hannah, where she practices integrative medicine, blending Western and Eastern approaches to patient care.

Dr. Aihan Kuhn

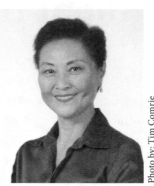

Photo by: Tim Comrie

A graduate of Hunan Medical University in China (now called Xiangya Medical School) in 1982, Dr. Aihan Kuhn has focused on holistic healing since 1992. During many years of practice, she has accumulated much experience with holistic medicine and achieved a great reputation for her patient care and education work. Her patients benefit from her many important tips for self-improvement in physical, emotional, and spiritual well-being, as well as the simple and easy healing exercises provided to enable them to participate in healing. Dr. Kuhn incorporates tai chi and qigong into her healing methodologies, changing the lives of those who have struggled for many years with no relief from conventional medicine. Dr. Kuhn offers many wellness programs, natural healing workshops, and professional training programs, such as tai chi instructor training certification courses, qigong instructor training certification courses, and wellness tui na therapy certification courses. These highly rated programs have produced many quality teachers and therapists. Dr. Kuhn is president of the Tai Chi and Qi Gong Healing Institute (www.TaiChiHealing.org), a nonprofit organization that promotes natural healing and prevention.

Dr. Kuhn lives with her husband Gerry Kuhn in Sarasota, Florida. For more information, please visit her website at www.draihankuhn.com.

BOOKS FROM YMAA

101 REFLECTIONS ON TAI CHI CHUAN
108 INSIGHTS INTO TAI CHI CHUAN
A SUDDEN DAWN: THE EPIC JOURNEY OF BODHIDHARMA
A WOMAN'S QIGONG GUIDE
ADVANCING IN TAE KWON DO
ANALYSIS OF SHAOLIN CHIN NA 2ND ED
ANCIENT CHINESE WEAPONS
THE ART AND SCIENCE OF STAFF FIGHTING
ART OF HOJO UNDO
ARTHRITIS RELIEF, 3D ED.
BACK PAIN RELIEF, 2ND ED.
BAGUAZHANG, 2ND ED.
BRAIN FITNESS
CARDIO KICKBOXING ELITE
CHIN NA IN GROUND FIGHTING
CHINESE FAST WRESTLING
CHINESE FITNESS
CHINESE TUI NA MASSAGE
CHOJUN
COMPREHENSIVE APPLICATIONS OF SHAOLIN CHIN NA
CONFLICT COMMUNICATION
CROCODILE AND THE CRANE: A NOVEL
CUTTING SEASON: A XENON PEARL MARTIAL ARTS THRILLER
DAO DE JING
DAO IN ACTION
DEFENSIVE TACTICS
DESHI: A CONNOR BURKE MARTIAL ARTS THRILLER
DIRTY GROUND
DR. WU'S HEAD MASSAGE
DUKKHA HUNGRY GHOSTS
DUKKHA REVERB
DUKKHA, THE SUFFERING: AN EYE FOR AN EYE
DUKKHA UNLOADED
ENZAN: THE FAR MOUNTAIN, A CONNOR BURKE MARTIAL ARTS
    THRILLER
ESSENCE OF SHAOLIN WHITE CRANE
EVEN IF IT KILLS ME
EXPLORING TAI CHI
FACING VIOLENCE
FIGHT BACK
FIGHT LIKE A PHYSICIST
THE FIGHTER'S BODY
FIGHTER'S FACT BOOK
FIGHTER'S FACT BOOK 2
THE FIGHTING ARTS
FIGHTING THE PAIN RESISTANT ATTACKER
FIRST DEFENSE
FORCE DECISIONS: A CITIZENS GUIDE
FOX BORROWS THE TIGER'S AWE
INSIDE TAI CHI
THE JUDO ADVANTAGE
THE JUJI GATAME ENCYCLOPEDIA
KAGE: THE SHADOW, A CONNOR BURKE MARTIAL ARTS THRILLER
KARATE SCIENCE
KATA AND THE TRANSMISSION OF KNOWLEDGE
KRAV MAGA PROFESSIONAL TACTICS
KRAV MAGA WEAPON DEFENSES
LITTLE BLACK BOOK OF VIOLENCE
LIUHEBAFA FIVE CHARACTER SECRETS
MARTIAL ARTS ATHLETE
MARTIAL ARTS INSTRUCTION
MARTIAL WAY AND ITS VIRTUES
MASK OF THE KING
MEDITATIONS ON VIOLENCE
MERIDIAN QIGONG EXERCISES
MIND/BODY FITNESS
MINDFUL EXERCISE
THE MIND INSIDE TAI CHI
THE MIND INSIDE YANG STYLE TAI CHI CHUAN
MUGAI RYU
NATURAL HEALING WITH QIGONG
NORTHERN SHAOLIN SWORD, 2ND ED.
OKINAWA'S COMPLETE KARATE SYSTEM: ISSHIN RYU
THE PAIN-FREE BACK

PAIN-FREE JOINTS
POWER BODY
PRINCIPLES OF TRADITIONAL CHINESE MEDICINE
THE PROTECTOR ETHIC
QIGONG FOR HEALTH & MARTIAL ARTS 2ND ED.
QIGONG FOR LIVING
QIGONG FOR TREATING COMMON AILMENTS
QIGONG MASSAGE
QIGONG MEDITATION: EMBRYONIC BREATHING
QIGONG MEDITATION: SMALL CIRCULATION
QIGONG, THE SECRET OF YOUTH: DA MO'S CLASSICS
QUIET TEACHER: A XENON PEARL MARTIAL ARTS THRILLER
RAVEN'S WARRIOR
REDEMPTION
ROOT OF CHINESE QIGONG, 2ND ED.
SCALING FORCE
SELF-DEFENSE FOR WOMEN
SENSEI: A CONNOR BURKE MARTIAL ARTS THRILLER
SHIHAN TE: THE BUNKAI OF KATA
SHIN GI TAI: KARATE TRAINING FOR BODY, MIND, AND SPIRIT
SIMPLE CHINESE MEDICINE
SIMPLE QIGONG EXERCISES FOR HEALTH, 3RD ED.
SIMPLIFIED TAI CHI CHUAN, 2ND ED.
SOLO TRAINING
SOLO TRAINING 2
SUMO FOR MIXED MARTIAL ARTS
SUNRISE TAI CHI
SUNSET TAI CHI
SURVIVING ARMED ASSAULTS
TAE KWON DO: THE KOREAN MARTIAL ART
TAEKWONDO BLACK BELT POOMSAE
TAEKWONDO: A PATH TO EXCELLENCE
TAEKWONDO: ANCIENT WISDOM FOR THE MODERN WARRIOR
TAEKWONDO: DEFENSE AGAINST WEAPONS
TAEKWONDO: SPIRIT AND PRACTICE
TAO OF BIOENERGETICS
TAI CHI BALL QIGONG: FOR HEALTH AND MARTIAL ARTS
TAI CHI BALL WORKOUT FOR BEGINNERS
THE TAI CHI BOOK
TAI CHI CHIN NA: THE SEIZING ART OF TAI CHI CHUAN,
    2ND ED.
TAI CHI CHUAN CLASSICAL YANG STYLE, 2ND ED.
TAI CHI CHUAN MARTIAL POWER, 3RD ED.
TAI CHI CONNECTIONS
TAI CHI DYNAMICS
TAI CHI FOR DEPRESSION
TAI CHI IN 10 WEEKS
TAI CHI QIGONG, 3RD ED.
TAI CHI SECRETS OF THE ANCIENT MASTERS
TAI CHI SECRETS OF THE WU & LI STYLES
TAI CHI SECRETS OF THE WU STYLE
TAI CHI SECRETS OF THE YANG STYLE
TAI CHI SWORD: CLASSICAL YANG STYLE, 2ND ED.
TAI CHI SWORD FOR BEGINNERS
TAI CHI WALKING
TAIJIQUAN THEORY OF DR. YANG, JWING-MING
TAO OF BIOENERGETICS
TENGU: THE MOUNTAIN GOBLIN, A CONNOR BURKE MARTIAL ARTS
    THRILLER
TIMING IN THE FIGHTING ARTS
TRADITIONAL CHINESE HEALTH SECRETS
TRADITIONAL TAEKWONDO
TRAINING FOR SUDDEN VIOLENCE
TRUE WELLNESS
THE WARRIOR'S MANIFESTO
WAY OF KATA
WAY OF KENDO AND KENJITSU
WAY OF SANCHIN KATA
WAY TO BLACK BELT
WESTERN HERBS FOR MARTIAL ARTISTS
WILD GOOSE QIGONG
WINNING FIGHTS
WISDOM'S WAY
XINGYIQUAN

DVDS FROM YMAA

ADVANCED PRACTICAL CHIN NA IN-DEPTH
ANALYSIS OF SHAOLIN CHIN NA
ATTACK THE ATTACK
BAGUA FOR BEGINNERS 1
BAGUAZHANG: EMEI BAGUAZHANG
BEGINNER QIGONG FOR WOMEN 1
BEGINNER QIGONG FOR WOMEN 2
CHEN STYLE TAIJIQUAN
CHEN TAI CHI FOR BEGINNERS
CHIN NA IN-DEPTH COURSES 1—4
CHIN NA IN-DEPTH COURSES 5—8
CHIN NA IN-DEPTH COURSES 9—12
FACING VIOLENCE: 7 THINGS A MARTIAL ARTIST MUST KNOW
FIVE ANIMAL SPORTS
FIVE ELEMENTS ENERGY BALANCE
INFIGHTING
INTRODUCTION TO QI GONG FOR BEGINNERS
JOINT LOCKS
KNIFE DEFENSE: TRADITIONAL TECHNIQUES AGAINST A DAGGER
KUNG FU BODY CONDITIONING 1
KUNG FU BODY CONDITIONING 2
KUNG FU FOR KIDS
KUNG FU FOR TEENS
LIANG TAI CHI FOR HEALTH
LOGIC OF VIOLENCE
MERIDIAN QIGONG
NEIGONG FOR MARTIAL ARTS
NORTHERN SHAOLIN SWORD : SAN CAI JIAN, KUN WU JIAN, QI MEN JIAN
QI GONG 30-DAY CHALLENGE
QI GONG FOR ANXIETY
QI GONG FOR ARMS, WRISTS, AND HANDS
QI GONG FOR BETTER BREATHING
QI GONG FOR CANCER
QI GONG FOR ENERGY AND VITALITY
QI GONG FOR HEADACHES
QI GONG FOR HEALING
QI GONG FOR HEALTHY JOINTS
QI GONG FOR HIGH BLOOD PRESSURE
QIGONG FOR LONGEVITY
QI GONG FOR STRONG BONES
QI GONG FOR THE UPPER BACK AND NECK
QIGONG FOR BEGINNERS
QIGONG FOR WOMEN
QIGONG FOR WOMEN WITH DAISY LEE
QIGONG MASSAGE
QIGONG MINDFULNESS IN MOTION
QIGONG: 15 MINUTES TO HEALTH
SABER FUNDAMENTAL TRAINING
SAI TRAINING AND SEQUENCES
SANCHIN KATA: TRADITIONAL TRAINING FOR KARATE POWER
SCALING FORCE
SHAOLIN KUNG FU FUNDAMENTAL TRAINING: COURSES 1 & 2
SHAOLIN LONG FIST KUNG FU: ADVANCED SEQUENCES 1
SHAOLIN LONG FIST KUNG FU: ADVANCED SEQUENCES 2
SHAOLIN LONG FIST KUNG FU: BASIC SEQUENCES
SHAOLIN LONG FIST KUNG FU: INTERMEDIATE SEQUENCES

SHAOLIN SABER: BASIC SEQUENCES
SHAOLIN STAFF: BASIC SEQUENCES
SHAOLIN WHITE CRANE GONG FU BASIC TRAINING: COURSES 1 &
SHAOLIN WHITE CRANE GONG FU BASIC TRAINING: COURSES 3 &
SHUAI JIAO: KUNG FU WRESTLING
SIMPLE QIGONG EXERCISES FOR HEALTH
SIMPLE QIGONG EXERCISES FOR ARTHRITIS RELIEF
SIMPLE QIGONG EXERCISES FOR BACK PAIN RELIEF
SIMPLIFIED TAI CHI CHUAN: 24 & 48 POSTURES
SIMPLIFIED TAI CHI FOR BEGINNERS 48
SUNRISE TAI CHI
SUNSET TAI CHI
SWORD: FUNDAMENTAL TRAINING
TAEKWONDO KORYO POOMSAE
TAI CHI BALL QIGONG: COURSES 1 & 2
TAI CHI BALL QIGONG: COURSES 3 & 4
TAI CHI BALL WORKOUT FOR BEGINNERS
TAI CHI CHUAN CLASSICAL YANG STYLE
TAI CHI CONNECTIONS
TAI CHI ENERGY PATTERNS
TAI CHI FIGHTING SET
TAI CHI FIT: 24 FORM
TAI CHI FIT: FLOW
TAI CHI FIT: FUSION BAMBOO
TAI CHI FIT: FUSION FIRE
TAI CHI FIT: FUSION IRON
TAI CHI FIT IN PARADISE
TAI CHI FIT: OVER 50
TAI CHI FIT: STRENGTH
TAI CHI FIT: TO GO
TAI CHI FOR WOMEN
TAI CHI FUSION: FIRE
TAI CHI QIGONG
TAI CHI PUSHING HANDS: COURSES 1 & 2
TAI CHI PUSHING HANDS: COURSES 3 & 4
TAI CHI SWORD: CLASSICAL YANG STYLE
TAI CHI SWORD FOR BEGINNERS
TAI CHI SYMBOL: YIN YANG STICKING HANDS
TAIJI & SHAOLIN STAFF: FUNDAMENTAL TRAINING
TAIJI CHIN NA IN-DEPTH
TAIJI 37 POSTURES MARTIAL APPLICATIONS
TAIJI SABER CLASSICAL YANG STYLE
TAIJI WRESTLING
TRAINING FOR SUDDEN VIOLENCE
UNDERSTANDING QIGONG 1: WHAT IS QI? • HUMAN QI
    CIRCULATORY SYSTEM
UNDERSTANDING QIGONG 2: KEY POINTS • QIGONG BREATHING
UNDERSTANDING QIGONG 3: EMBRYONIC BREATHING
UNDERSTANDING QIGONG 4: FOUR SEASONS QIGONG
UNDERSTANDING QIGONG 5: SMALL CIRCULATION
UNDERSTANDING QIGONG 6: MARTIAL QIGONG BREATHING
WHITE CRANE HARD & SOFT QIGONG
WUDANG KUNG FU: FUNDAMENTAL TRAINING
WUDANG SWORD
WUDANG TAIJIQUAN
XINGYIQUAN
YANG TAI CHI FOR BEGINNERS

more products available from . . .
YMAA Publication Center, Inc. 楊氏東方文化出版中心
1-800-669-8892 • info@ymaa.com • www.ymaa.com